Jungle Tales

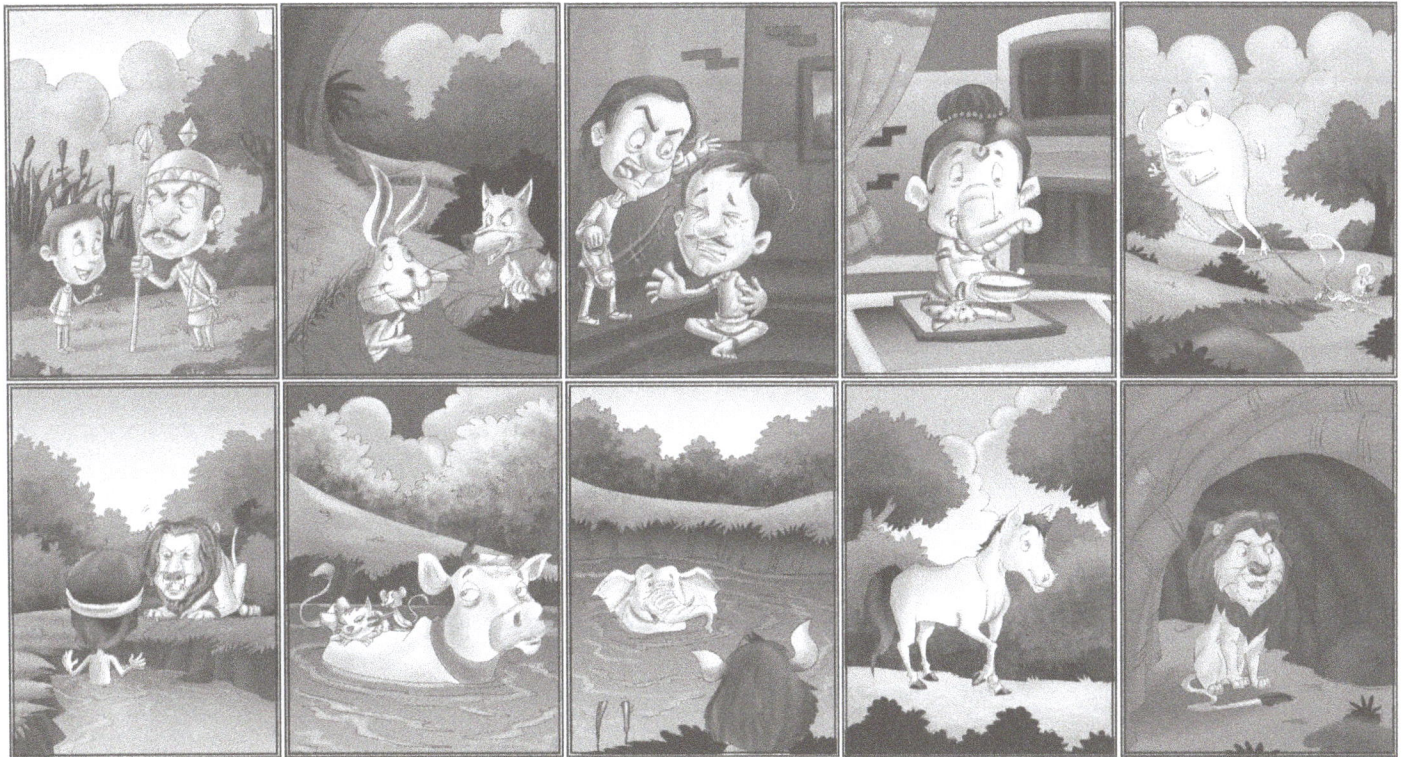

GOPU
BOOKS

An Imprint of V&S PUBLISHERS

Published by:

G❍PU
BOOKS

An Imprint of V&S PUBLISHERS

F-2/16, Ansari Road, Daryaganj, New Delhi-110002
011-23240026, 011-23240027 • *Fax:* 011-23240028
Email: info@vspublishers.com • *Website:* www.vspublishers.com

Regional Office : Hyderabad
5-1-707/1, Brij Bhawan (Beside Central Bank of India Lane)
Bank Street, Koti, Hyderabad - 500 095
040-24737290
E-mail: vspublishershyd@gmail.com

Follow us on: 🇹 🇫 in

For any assistance sms **VSPUB** to **56161**

All books available at **www.vspublishers.com**

Printed at : Param Offseters, Okhla, New Delhi-110020

publisher's notes

V&S Publishers has been in the forefront in publishing story books for children - under the imprint Gopu Books. Most books are educational, moral and value-based in nature. Nearly every book published under this imprint has been lapped up by parents and guardians on behalf of their children, both in English and Hindi versions. Since the dawn of time, parents have used stories with morals to teach children about the values of the family, about life, difference between right and wrong, good and bad. A story with a moral can help, more so contemporary ones with which children can relate conveniently. Unlike most prevalent books in the market that exist only for their entertainment value, this book **Jungle Tales for Children** offers to build strength of character and respect for others.

This book is a compilation of 50 one-page stories for children. Language used is elementary and simple. Each story comes with caricature based illustration in black & white – a presentation no other publisher has attempted before. Being different from the ordinary run of the mills type, the caricatures retain interest of young readers. The moral at the end of the story summaries precisely what the child is supposed to learn!

By reading stories, children will gather how characters deal with situations and work through issues, they gain experience without having to go through those conditions themselves. Their horizon is expanded that fits the ethos and mores of a traditional society like ours.

We would be glad to receive feedback from parents so that future publications retain the flavour of enlightened views that expand horizon of our young readers.

----

contents

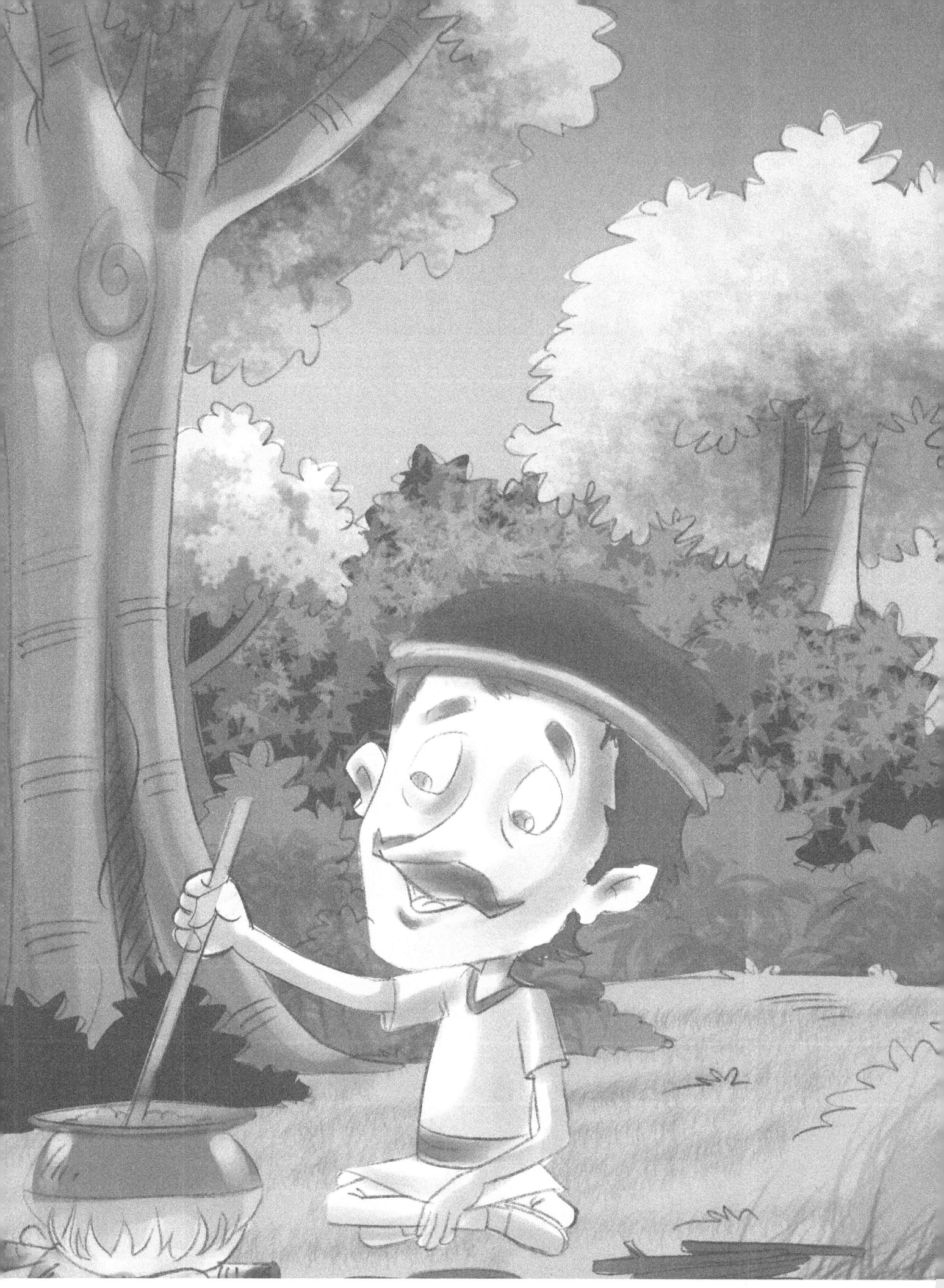

reward for a mindless fool

*R*amlal got his son married. In order to carry his dowry his son's in laws gave him several donkeys. But one donkey was a prankster. He would trot and hop around all the time. Therefore Ramlal decided to leave him half way through. And the donkey lived independently in the jungles. One day a man on bullock cart arrived in the jungle. He sat under a shady tree to rest for a while. He tied his bulls from a tree and started to cook a meal for himself.

Donkey went on trotting towards those bulls. He said, 'if you will listen to me I can free you from this painful job of bearing burden.' But both the bulls were related, one was the uncle and other was the nephew. The uncle bull liked what the donkey has suggested here, whereas the nephew bull shrugged the donkey's suggestion off. He said, 'our master keeps us so well why you don't see that.' Donkey replied, 'after all you are a slave.' And the uncle bull decided to follow this donkey's advice from the time on. As soon as the bullock cart started to move the uncle bull fell on the ground flat. And started to breathe heavily.

The bullock cart driver thought his bull has fallen ill. But how can he drag his cart with only one bull? He looked around in the forest and saw a donkey was roaming there. The driver did not see here or there he caught hold of the donkey and dragged him in his cart to be pulled. And lugged the ill uncle bull over his bullock cart. To see donkey working at the place of a bull, the nephew bull remarked, 'this is what happens to those who try to work and advice mindlessly.'

Moral

What one does, gets it back this is the teaching of time.

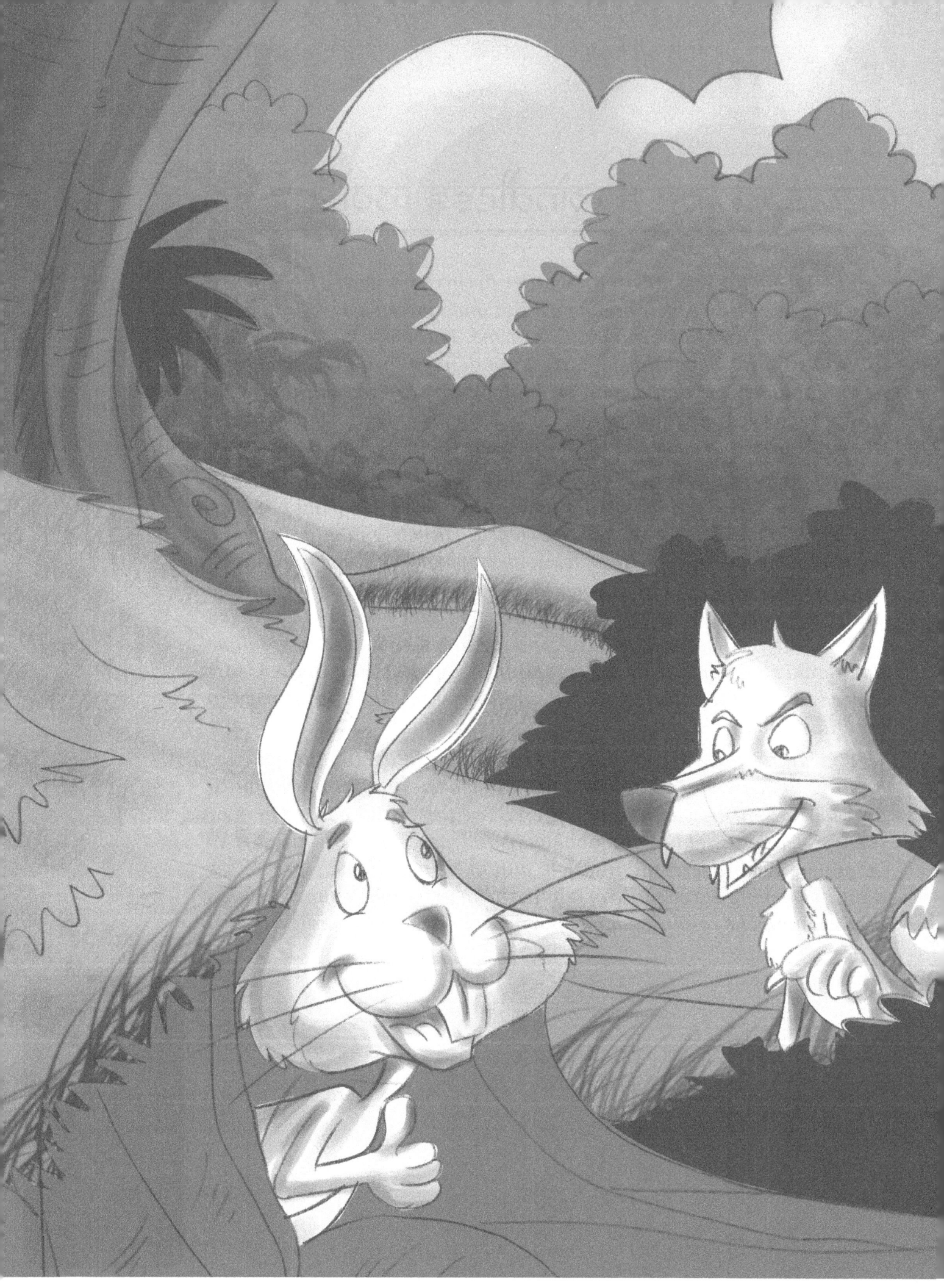

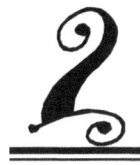

the tug of privilege

*O*nce upon a time there was a forest. In that forest there lived a Fox. She used to think very clever of herself. One day a rabbit came running and hid himself in her burrow. The fox asked, 'why did you come running here and have put your life in danger as well.' The rabbit held his breath calmly and spoke after hiding his fear, 'Oh dear sister! All the animals in the jungle are after my life to take over the post of jungle chief. But I do not intend to become one. And after a lot of struggle I just ran away by avoiding there persuasions.'

Fox replied, 'are you a fool? To be a chief is the matter of privilege and it has its own charm as well. If one has power in one's hand then what can be better than that.' Rabbit said, 'then why don't you take this position sister? I cannot possibly take care of this position on my own.' Fox was very pleased and somewhat greedy of getting such a powerful position, as soon as she went outside to grab hold of the position, she saw two blood thirsty tigers waiting for the rabbit to arrive. They both pounced at the fox. Somehow she escaped but in this ordeal both of her ears were eaten by the tigers and they snatched it. Fox ran inside her burrow and this time rabbit asked, 'why dear sister you have come so soon?' the fox replied, 'there is a lot of hassle in being the jungle chief, so much so that it can cost you your ears.' To become a ruler without having the right ability brings such misery to people who aspire for bigger positions in life.

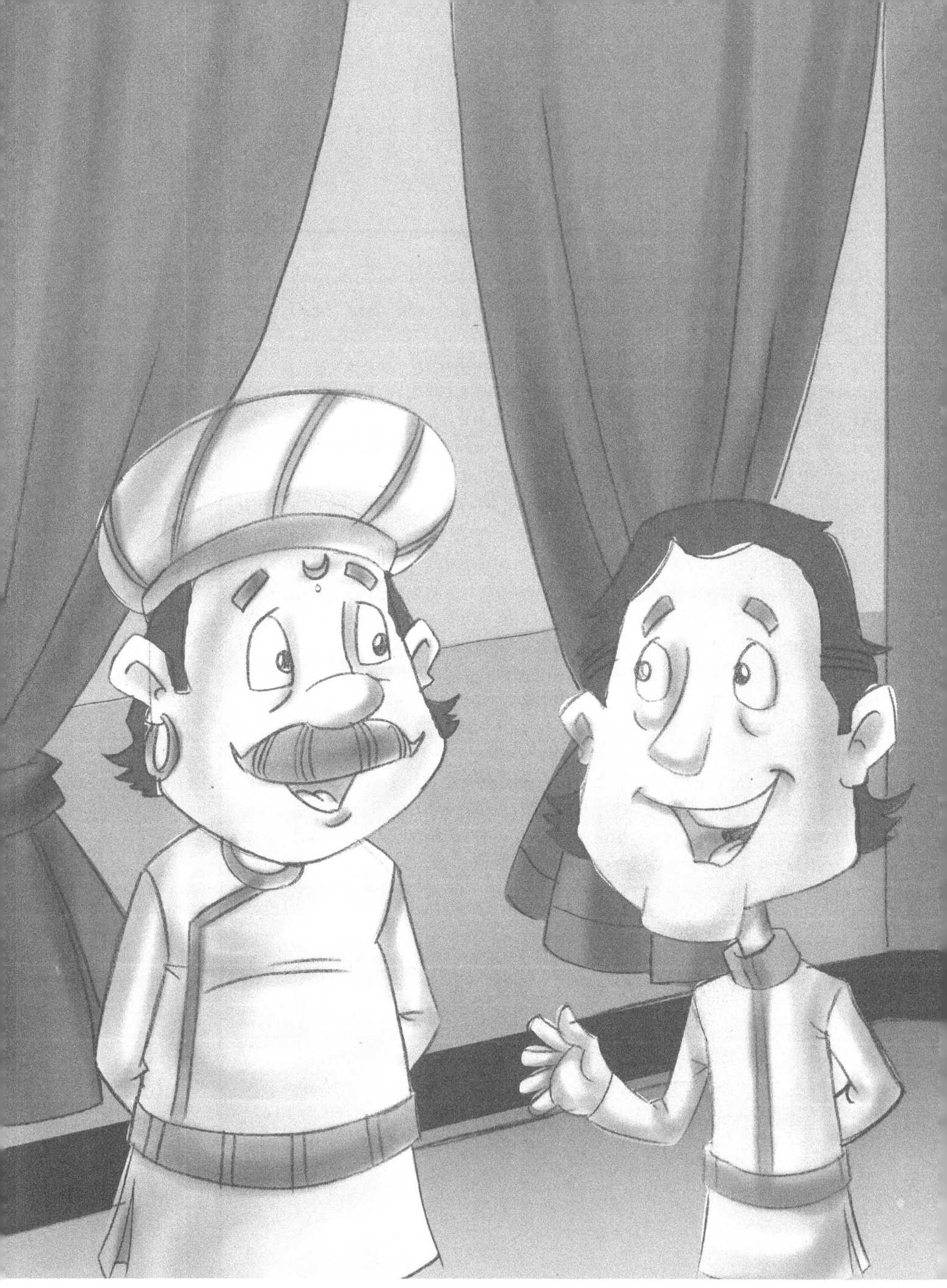

the golden horse

In Shivpur village there lived a man called Manik. Whatever Manik had to say he will elongate it till length. To spin yarns was one of his habits. One day Manik was sitting outside his house. All of a sudden King's men came looking for something there. They asked him if he has seen a white coloured horse passing by. But Manik was helpless because of his habit and said, 'the one who has seen a golden horse why he would be bothered to see a silver horse?' whatever Manik spoke all the King's men went and told this to their King, that one of his country person owns a gold coloured horse and such a horse can only be suitable for a king.

Manik was called immediately by the King. King said to Manik that he must give his golden horse to him and in return he can get as much gold as he wants from his treasure. But Manik was helpless by his own folly of blabbering; he said 'what I will do with so much of gold because I have seen heaps of diamonds myself.' But King asked Manik to take as much of diamond from him but he must give his golden horse to the him. But again Manik was busy spinning yarns and replied to the King, what I will do with all these diamonds I have seen several treasures of precious gems and jewels.

Again King said 'you can take as many precious jewels from me but give me your golden horse'. And Manik spoke again, 'what is gold or pearls and jewels or diamond or even a golden horse, which is nothing in worth because I have seen a flying horse as well'. Everyone understood by now Manik has a habit of spinning really long yarns and blabbering. In the end King got angry with him and asked, 'have you ever seen a dark dungeon or prison ever?' Manik was petrified after hearing about imprisonment and folded both his hands in front of the King in forgiveness. King took pity on him and spared him by from going to prison showing mercy. And Manik's gave up the nasty habit after having this ordeal in life.

Excessive blabbering and lying can put a person in life threatening situations.

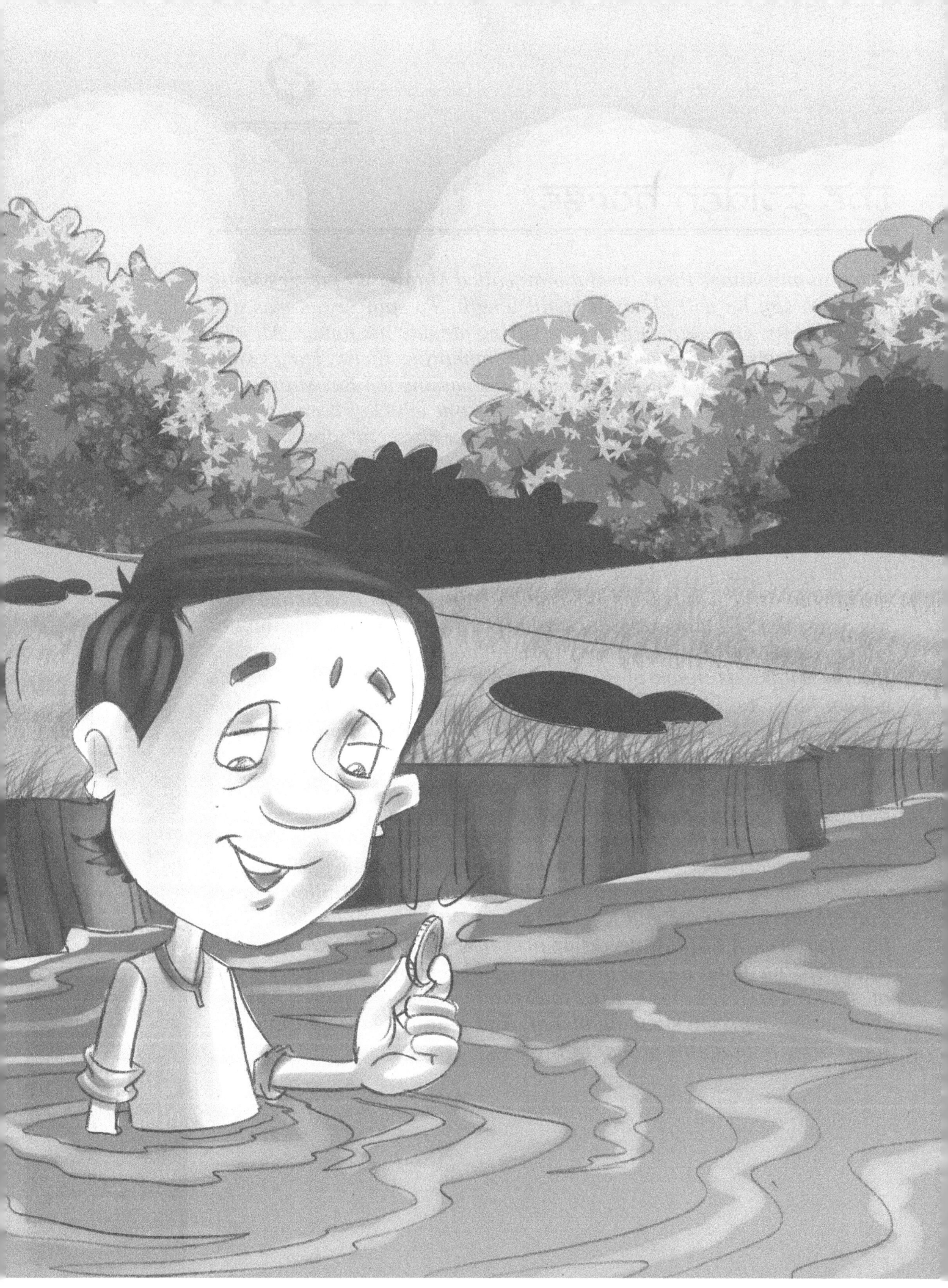

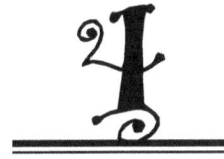

prowess of lion

Right across the bow of Mansarovar there came a swan flying every day. Swan would swim in the cool water of this lake and he used to dry itself while sitting on the shores. Near this lake there was a temple. A man named Bhola used to come to this temple to offer his prayers to the God. While coming and going he would pay his respect to the reverend lake's swan. In return the swan used to give him a gold coin every day. This went on for few days continuously but one day, from the nearby forest there came a lion to drink water on the bow of Mansarovar lake. Seeing the lion, swan got petrified and flew away and on the same spot where swan used to sit a crow came and took his position.

That day when Bhola was going towards the lake after praying in the temple, a priest stopped him and asked, 'where are you going brother?' He replied 'on the bank of Mansarovar a swan comes there. I go there to meet that swan every day. We have become quite fond of each other, till I see him or meet him I do not feel satisfied. He gives me a gold coin every day which I distribute amongst poor people equally.'

After listening to all this priest took a cold sigh and said, 'A crow is the head of the bow and the swan is gone, now it is where the lion lives and you must go your home now.' Which means a lion has made his home on the lake, on the place where swan sat now a crow sits there, therefore do not go to the lake anymore because lion might kill you as well. Bhola saw from a distance that this priest was right. The time has changed now. Instead of swan one could hear croaking sounds of a crow echoing on Mansarovar lake. Bhola understood it is better to go back home finally. He decided to change himself and move with the time.

Moral

Time is ever changing. It is considered always wise to walk with time and change accordingly.

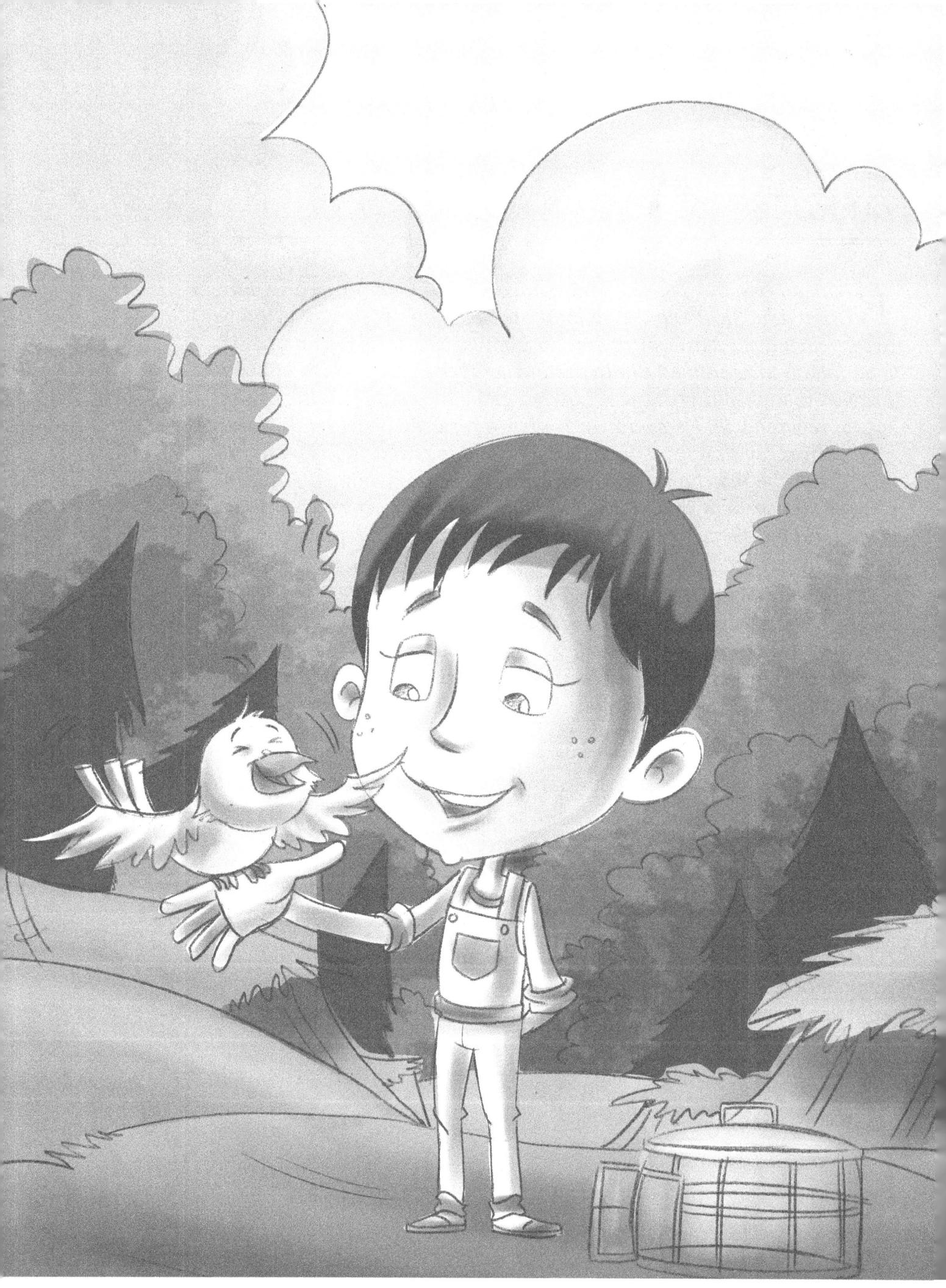

ā kind hearted boy

*T*here was a village in France where lived a boy whose name was Jean. He loved forest birds the most. He could know a bird by the sound it makes. One day while he was going someplace, suddenly he heard the sound of a bird. He sensed that the bird's voice was quite sad. After reaching a certain distance he met a man who had caged a bird. Jean knew that people like to eat this bird because they like the flesh of this particular bird. That is why anyone who will buy this bird will kill it to eat.

Jean went to the bird seller and asked what its cost was, and then he tried to fondle things inside his pocket. He had no sufficient money with him. Jean told the bird seller 'keep this money with you. I have bought this bird from you now. But I need some more money as a proper amount I will go and get it for you now. Do not sell this bird to anyone.' He ran towards his own house. He saw his mother had left for somewhere. What can be done now? He feared if he would delay someone else would buy that bird and will take it with him. And that bird's life will be in danger.

While standing there he remembered about his teacher. On a very hot scorching summer he went running to see his teacher. Within no time he told entire story to his teacher. The teacher was very kind hearted and he gave him money immediately. He did not stay for another moment there and went running to the place where the bird was; he saw another person was bargaining for the cost of the same bird. Jean paid the remaining money and took the bird inside the cage and bought it home. When he reached his head started spinning due to excessive heat. When he felt little better he first went near the cage and started kissing that bird with a lot of love. The bird also got happy and started fluttering its wings and showed its gratitude. Then Jean went out of his home to a desolate place where no one was and he took the bird's cage along. Jean freed the bird in open. Before flying away the bird turned toward him to have a final look of Jean out of so much love and adoration, and it flew away in the open sky forever.

Moral

There is no pleasure bigger than giving someone the gift of life.

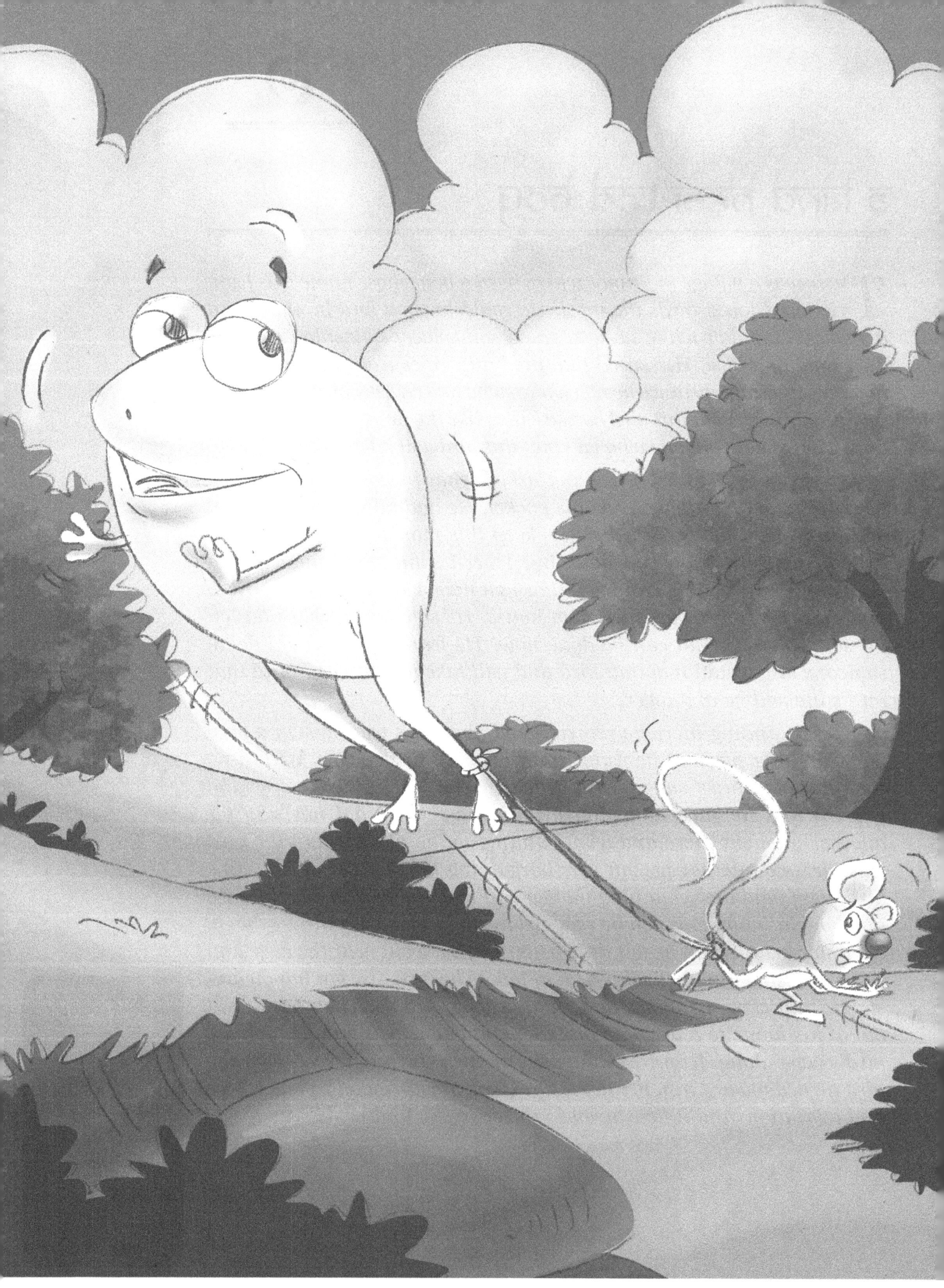

enmity of a friend

*O*nce upon a time there was a mouse and a frog. They were great friends. Every day the frog will come out from his pond and will go to see his friend mouse who lived under a tree. The frog would spend the day with his friend and in the evening he would return back to his pond again. The mouse was very pleased by the frog's friendship that he did not recognise how his friend had turned into his enemy by now. The reason for this enmity was very minute. Frog used to think that he comes to his friend's place every day to meet him but mouse never came to frog's house to see him not even once.

This matter pricked him a lot. He decided to avenge his friend mouse for this reason. One day when he was about to return from mouse's house he tied a string with one of his leg and its other end he tied with the mouse's tail and he started jumping. Poor mouse was dragged with the frog without his will and he kept on asking frog what the matter was. The frog did not reply at all and dived into the pond. Mouse tried real hard to escape but he was unable to and drowned in the pond.

After his death mouse's body was floating on the surface of water. When the eagle flying high in the sky saw the dead mouse floating on the water. It came flying low towards him picked the mouse with its beak and flew away. The string was tied to the frog's foot from the other end therefore the frog also came out of the water with a jerk. He tried to free himself but the eagle destroyed all his efforts. 'It is always said that never dig a trench for someone else because chances are one can tumble down in it oneself.'

If you try to dig a well for someone else, it is likely that you would become a victim by falling into it.

Never think of taking revenge. Leave such decisions to God who will take action He thanks best.

Moral

When someone desires wrong for somebody may land up as victim to his own folly.

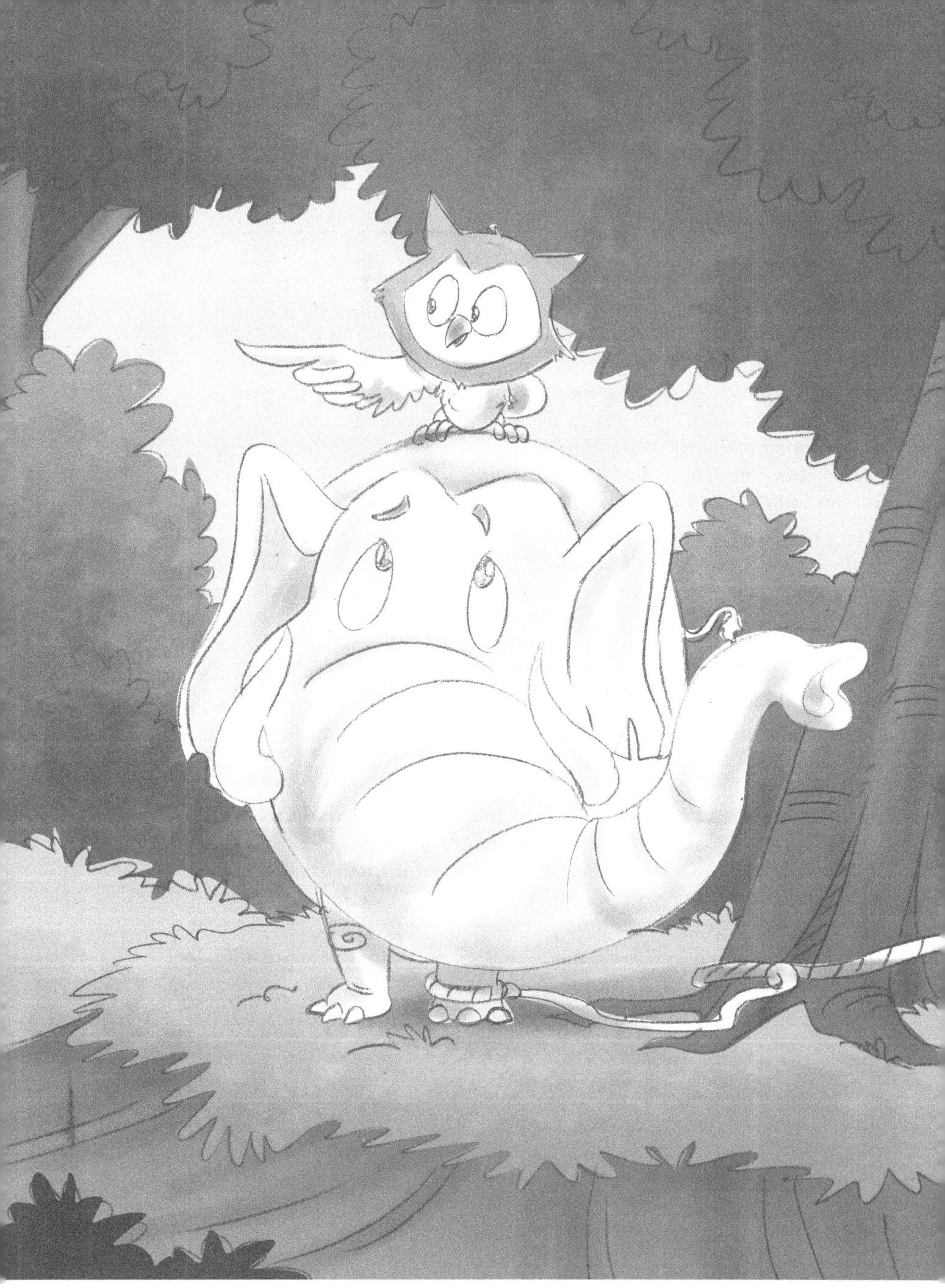

ā dream

There was a tree on which lived an owl. And right under that tree an elephant used to come at night to rest. Slowly they became good friends. One day in search of food elephant lost his way and he entered a feast organised by ogres. To have seen this elephant the king of all ogres screamed, 'oh it is this it is this!'

King's service men asked 'who is he Your Majesty?' The King of Ogres said, 'last night I had a dream. In which I was having a banquet made of an elephant. This elephant appears just what I saw in my dreams.'

'Catch him I will eat it so that my dream comes true.' All the Ogres got hold of the elephant. The elephant was so scared that he did not even try to free himself from the ogres. They tied the legs of this elephant. Then the king of ogres came with his queen right in front of elephant. And when the elephant did not return to that tree the owl came flying searching right under the tree where the ogres hadtied him. When he came flying under that tree he heard everything and the owl got to know what the entire affair was.

He started screaming, 'oh it is this, it is this'. While saying this he sat on the elephant's head. The king of all ogres asked the passing owl, 'what are you talking about?' owl said, I was talking about your queen. I had a dream last night that I have married your queen. So let me marry your queen so that my dream comes true.' The queen of the ogres was petrified after listening this. 'How can I marry an owl?' she said. After listening to her the king spoke, 'but no one is asking you to marry an owl.'

'It was just a dream. And who takes a dream so seriously?' the ogre king said further, 'see I have eaten this same elephant in my dream but now I am releasing him to go back.' After listening to him the elephant got freed and ran from there. He thanked his friend for his brave efforts.

Moral

Dreams are never true and authentic, one must never trust them.

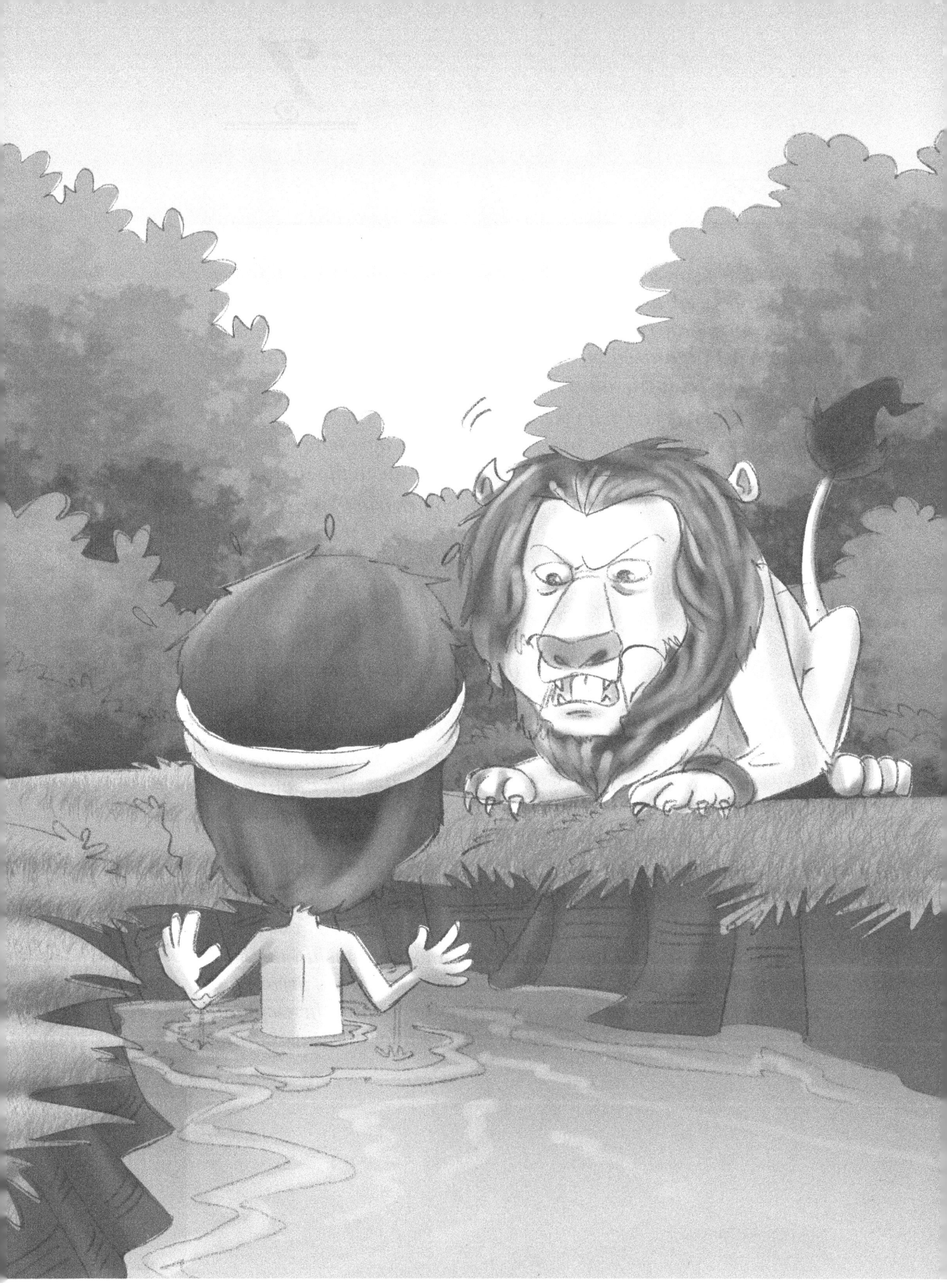

the misfortune of greed

*O*nce upon a time near a lake an old lion was sitting. He was unable to hunt his prey, but still he was a very clever creature. He had a gold bracelet. He would show this golden bracelet to passing by people and say, 'come close to me and take this bracelet with you because I want to give it away.' But because of fear no one wanted to come closer to him. One day a passer-by was crossing from there. After listening to this lion he thought all his life he was a poor man, 'if I will get this golden bracelet, I can spend rest of my life comfortably. But suddenly the thought crossed his mind what if to get that bracelet he lands up losing his precious life.'

After a lot of thought he asked the lion, 'yes it is right that you have this golden bracelet, but why should I trust you? If I will come closer to you to accept this golden bracelet and what if you gulp me down?' after listening to this the lion replied, 'your doubting me is justified because I am a lion, you can be unsure of me knowing I have killed a lot of innocent beings. Now I am old and want to correct my ways by doing charity so that I can be granted a better life next time. That is why do not think too much. You may come here have a pleasant bath in this lake and take this gold bracelet away.'

The passer-by was full of greed to what lion has told him. As soon as he went into the water he got stuck in the marshy surface of this lake. He struggled with his hand and feet but all his efforts were wasted. After seeing him worked up, the lion smiled and said, 'Oh poor you got stuck in marshland. But worry not I will take you out now.' By now passer-by understood that it was a big mistake to have trusted the lion. Before he could think of something else the lion took his life in one strike.

It is wise to think carefully before deciding to trust or not to trust someone whose character is doubtful. But the best idea is to avoid all such people. Greed always ends in disaster.

Moral

Greed is big vice. Never fall in its trap.

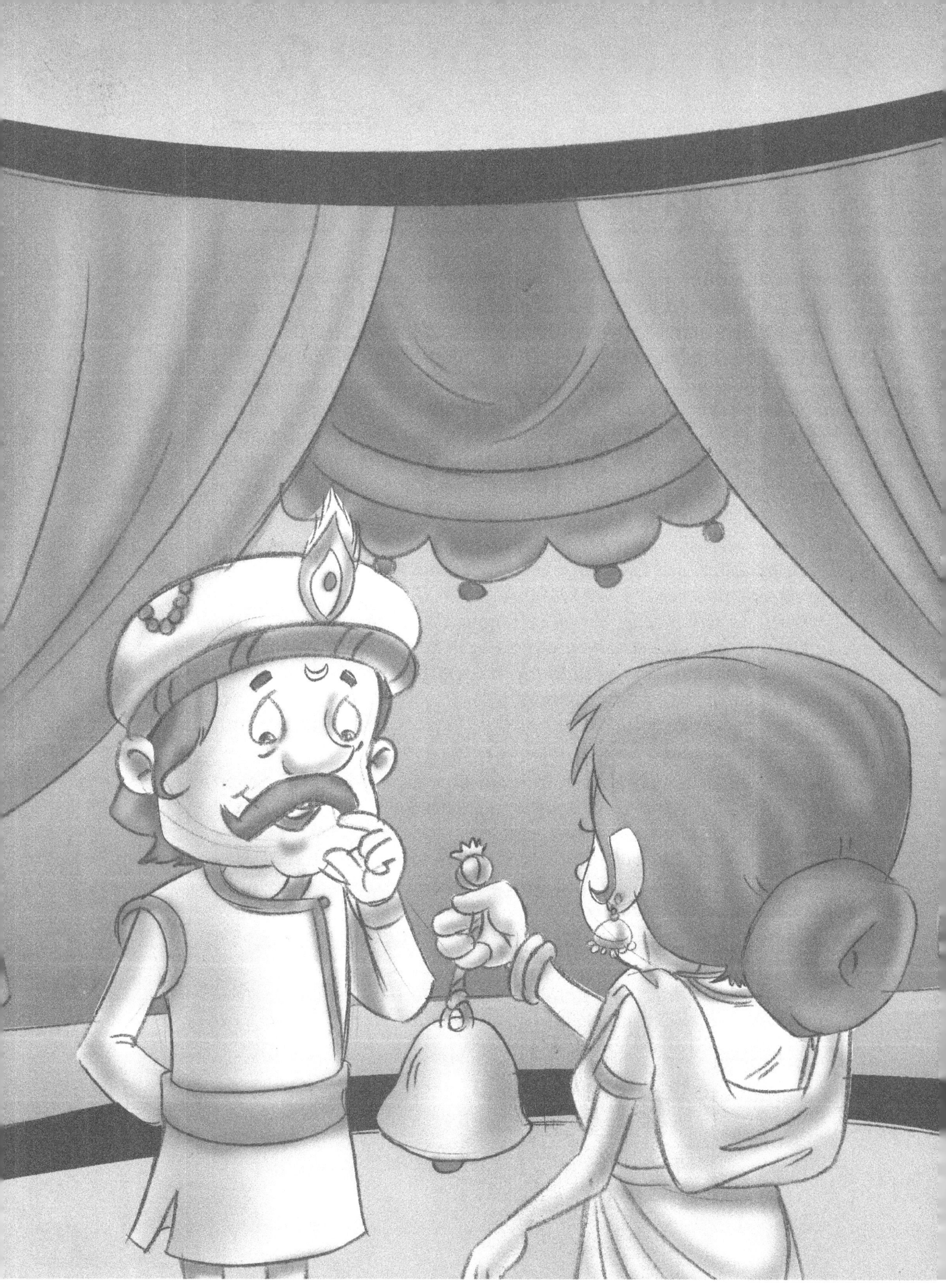

the end of a monster

*R*ight within Sriparbat there was a city called Brahmapura. Close by there was a dense forest. Long ago a thief had stolen a huge bell and he was running across this forest. A tiger saw him running. It attacked and killed the man. That bell remained there. Some monkeys came and lifted that bell. They would make it ring now and then. For people of Brahmapura that sound became a huge mystery. Some men gathered courage and went to the forest. They saw a half-eaten human body and heard nonstop ringing of the bell. They got scared and ran away from that forest to the city.

There they informed others that there lived a monster in the forest whose name is 'Bell-trotter'. He eats up human beings and then rings a bell. All the citizens of Brahmapura became terrified and started to leave this city one by one. In that very city there lived a woman named Karala. She thought why would a monster ring a bell. She thought there is a secret behind all this. One day she decided to go inside the forest. She saw a huge pack of monkeys. One of the monkeys from the same pack was ringing a huge bell. When she saw this she understood everything and returned back to meet the king of this city. She said to the king, 'Your majesty if you give me some money, I will control this monster known as 'Bell-Trotter' immediately.' Karala took the money from the king and came home. On her way back she bought all the fruits which monkeys liked.

Next day she carried all these fruits and went straight to the forest. Even then she could hear bell ringing continuously. She followed the sound of this bell and reached near the pack of monkeys. When she reached on the spot Karala scattered all the fruits on the ground. To see fruits scattered on the ground all monkeys climbed down and dropped that huge bell on the ground. This is what Karala wanted to happen. She picked that bell and reached the king's court and spoke, 'Here is the bell of the 'Bell- Trotter' monster. I have nailed down that monster now.' Seeing Karala's valour the king rewarded her with a lot of gifts.

Moral

Every good work is always rewarded

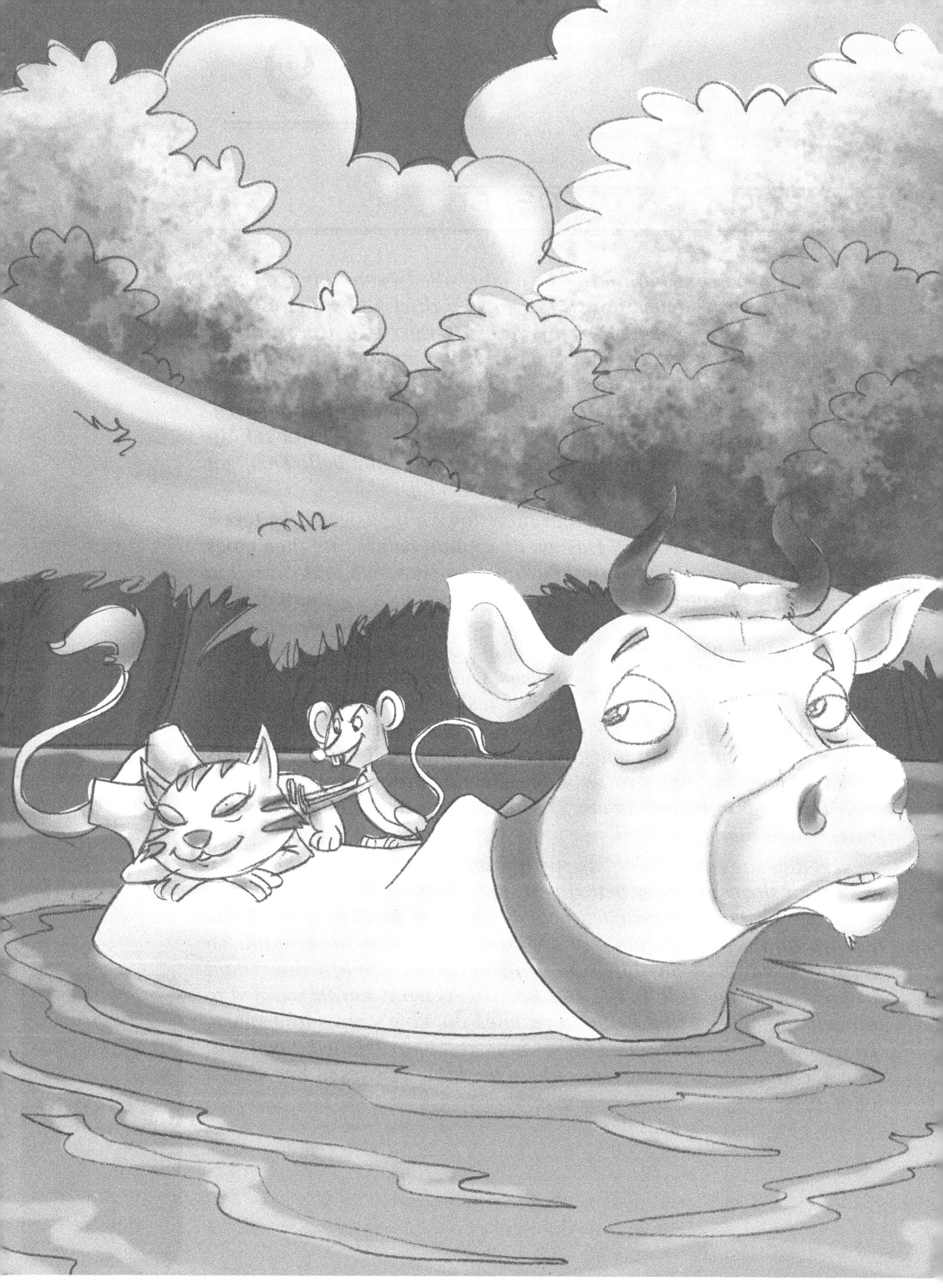

cat and the mouse

Long, long time ago, an emperor of China called Jade organised a tournament for animals in his kingdom. According to this tournament which was a race all the first twelve position holding animals will be given a certain value and place in their astronomical calendar and it was decided that, an entire year will be named after them. The cat and the mouse also wanted to participate in this tournament as well, but there was one major problem. They both could not wake up early in the morning. That is why they both requested their common friend, the bull to wake them early in the morning on the day of this tournament. Bull tried to wake them early morning real hard but it was of no use. The time for the race was about to begin. The bull did not want to leave them there. So he picked up both of them on his back and started running. The mouse woke up when Bull was at the last stage of his race which was when he was crossing the river. The mouse was very clever he knew that he could never win a race with cat. He tried to use his good luck today when he found out a better opportunity he pushed cat from the bull's back. As soon as the bull crossed the river and came out of the water the mouse leapt from his back and ran as hurriedly as he could and went ahead of him in the race and won it too. Lion was also given third position in this race and he had also cheated to win it. He kept his feet on other animal that is why lion also won a rank in the race.

This is the reason why in Chinese astronomical calendar the year starts with the year of 'Mouse'. And then there is the place for Bull and then comes the Lion. After them come Rabbit, Dragon, Snake, Horse, Goat, Monkey, Rooster, Dog and Pig in this calendar. And the cat has no place in this entire calendar. It was not amongst the first twelve animals that won this race. But somehow cat saved itself from getting drowned in the river. There is no doubt that the cat is till date chasing the mouse, because somewhere the cat has not forgotten what insult has been done by mouse on its ancestors.

It is true that more than hard labour, it is intelligence that wins the day.

Moral

Any work done by valour and brains will always gets recognised.

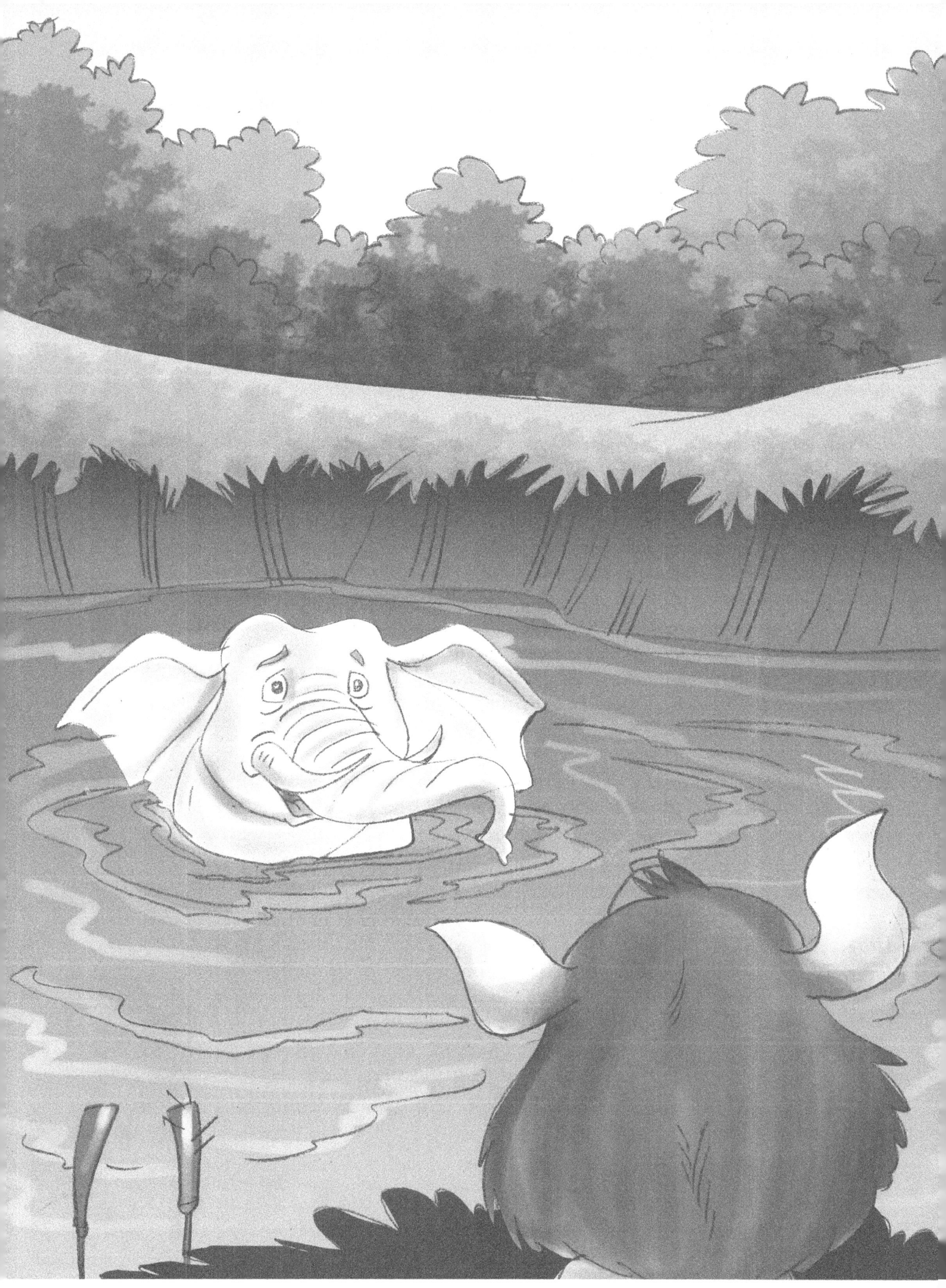

ā ẅicked jāckāl

There was an elephant which lived in the forests of Brahmavana. After seeing him a jackal thought, if I will kill this giant elephant then I can have food to eat throughout the month. But jackal could not understand how he could hunt such a big animal on his own. There was an old jackal in his pack, who spoke 'with my brain and power I can hunt that elephant down.'

The old jackal took the younger one in full confidence and went to see the elephant and said, 'Kindly accept my life. I have come to you in order to make an earnest request.' Elephant asked him 'what do you want to say?' to that old jackal said, 'all the animals have decided in this forest to make you as the head of this jungle.' After learning this fact elephant grew very happy.

Old jackal told him to be crowned as the king of the jungle the auspicious time was about to start from now, that is why he was needed to bath and start as soon as possible. After listening to him elephant went ahead with that wicked jackal immediately. Elephant did not even bother to think why all animals from the animal kingdom have sent only such a deceitful and wicked creature alone. The jackal got him close to the lake, which was extremely marshy. As soon as elephant went inside the lake to bath he got stuck into the marshy water. As much as he would try to free himself from it he would get stuck even more due to his heavy body. He got panicked and said to jackal, 'what should I do now my dear friend jackal? Help me out of this marshy water.'

Jackal laughed and spoke, 'No I will not help you out from this place because why did you trust me and agre to come with me? After a lot of effort elephant could not manage to come out of the marsh and died there after being stuck in it badly. After that all the wicked jackals feasted on the dead elephant's corpse.

It is said that friendship blossoms only amongst equals. You must be very cautious while developing friendship with new people. You must also try to understand why the other person is being extra nice to befriend you.

Moral

One must never trust a wicked minded person ever.

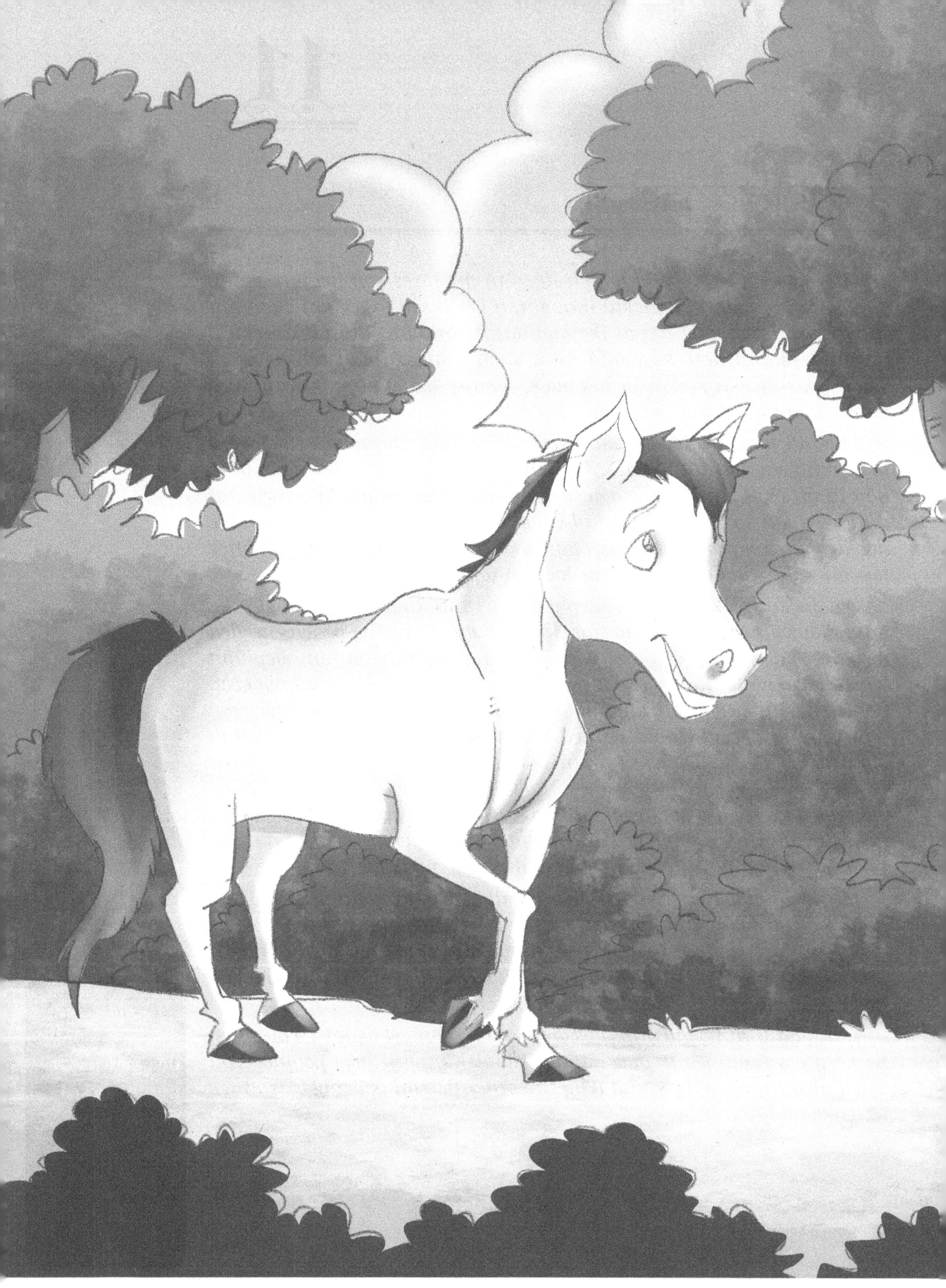

desiring to be beautiful

*O*nce upon a time long ago. God had a horse. It was very beautiful and hale and hearty to look at. It was also God's favourite horse too. Even after all this the horse was not satisfied with itself. The horse desired to be more beautiful. One day horse asked God, 'Dear Lord! You have made me very beautiful. And you loved and adored me as well. Now I derive you to make me more beautiful. So that I will be more grateful to you forever.'

God said 'I agree to make you even more beautiful. Now tell me what changes you want to have in you?' horse spoke 'my body is not proportionate. My neck is so small. If it is possible make it longer so that my upper body appears pleasing to look at. Also make my legs more thinner and longer so that they look better.' Then God said, 'So be it!' and the horse started looking like a camel. To see what has happened the horse got worried with his looks and started crying. He said 'Oh dear Lord! I wanted to become more handsome what did you do?' God replied 'this is what you wanted to look like, now you are a camel. And this is what you chose.'

Horse said while crying, 'but no I do not want to become a camel. As a horse every one found me beautiful but as a camel no one will like me.' Then God said 'whatever I gave you remain happy in that. You must not aim to receive more. This will create greed in you to acquire more and more. This can create problems for you which you may not be able to bear. Everything which I have created in this world has its own beauty. A camel is not as handsome as you but still it has no desire for more vanity. A camel can bear heavy burden and it understands its responsibility while being satisfied with his life.' Horse pleaded in front of God 'now I understand! Kindly turn me into a horse again.' And God did make him a horse again.

It is truly said that God has created everything with certain objective in mind. Every creation of God is useful in one way or the other.

To become greedy almost always ends in disaster. So be happy with what you are and what you have.

Moral

God has never created anything ugly. Everything created by him has some good quality or the other.

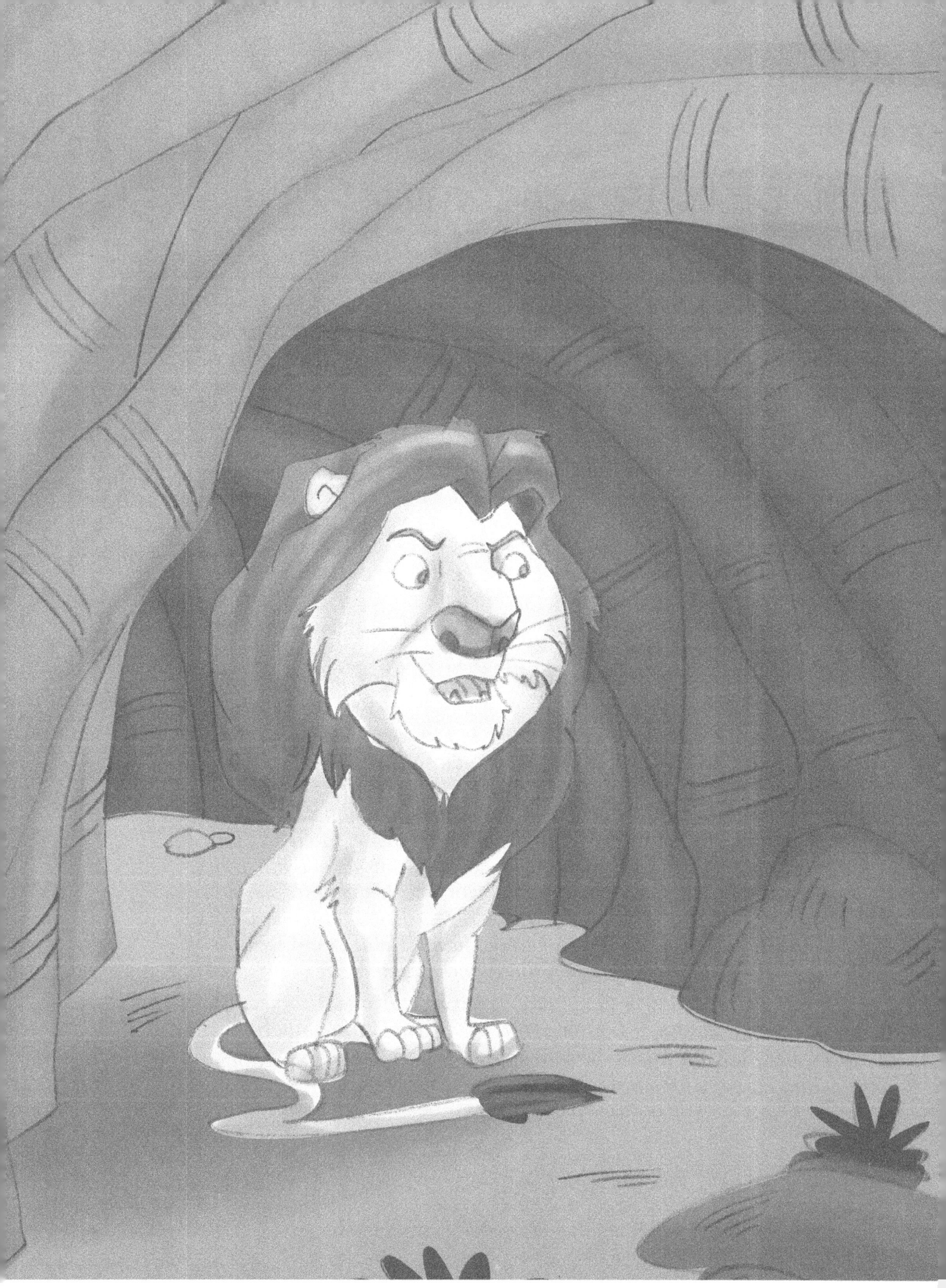

mean lion

*I*n the Northern Province there was a mountain it was known as 'Aburd'. Right below that mountain there was a cave, in which lived a lion. When at night the lion used to be in deep sleep there came a mouse all tip toed and he would bite the hair from his manes towards his neck. And when the lion would wake up next morning and would see his bad hair he would get angry, but he was helpless, because the mouse would be out of his reach by then. He would keep on thinking how to get his small enemy in his clutches? One day he left the forest to go towards the village. There he saw an otter. Somehow lion convinced him to come with him in his cave. He really welcomed and treated him nicely in his cave. The otter was very pleased with the lion and started to live with him in his cave.

One day mouse learnt that an enemy of his has come to live inside this cave, since then he stopped to come to the cave at night. Now lion was also at ease and slept well during the nights. Whenever he could hear mouse's voice he would serve even better meat to the otter so that due to the greed of getting better meat otter would live there. And this otter was living without any worry regarding his food. One day lion went outside to hunt for food and otter was in the cave. As soon as the lion went outside the mouse came out looking for his own food. Suddenly the otter saw the mouse. Then what could happen more, he jumped and clutched him immediately and gulped the mouse down without a thought.

When lion did not hear this mouse's voice for a long time, he understood that otter has made him his prey finally. Now lion was at peace. And when there was no mouse in the cave then he did not need otter there to live with him. He started to disregard the otter since then. Sometimes he would give him food and sometimes he won't. Due to the fear the otter could not even complain about it. He grew frail day by day and one day he died because of hunger.

Moral

Togetherness of a similar kind is healthy. The friendship or enmity with a mightier person is never good.

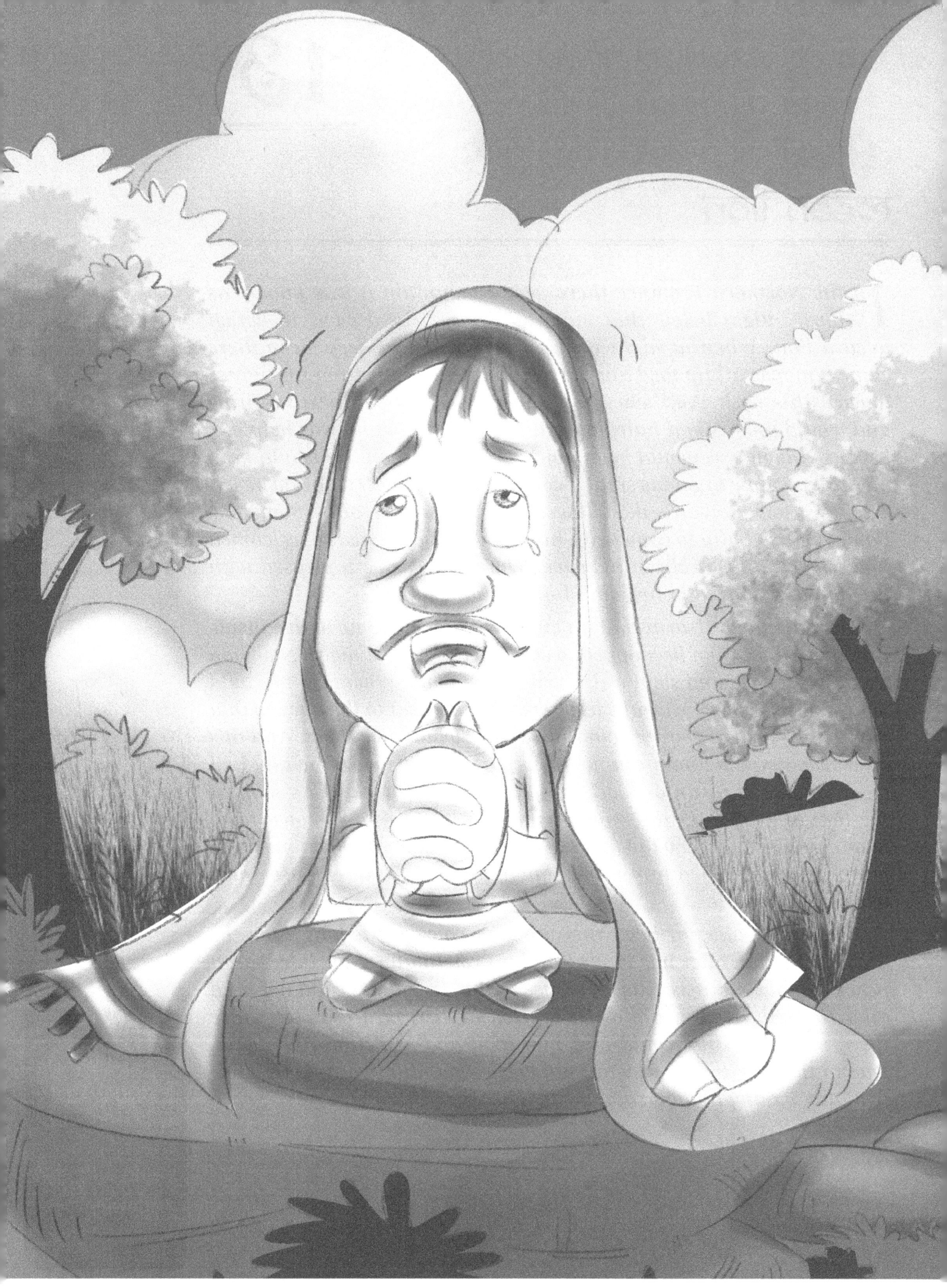

buffalo's grazing

*I*n a village a man named Birji lived. All day long he would take all cattle for grazing and when evening fell would bring them back home. It was winter times. And Birji's cattle were grazing around the forest. Birji was cloaked inside a blanket and he was lying on a big stone nearby. While lying down he fell asleep. He slept there peacefully. When he got up he started to count his cattle and found out a buffalo was missing from there. Now Birji was worried. The owner of the buffalo was Thakur. When he learned about his missing buffalo he became angry. He wondered the Thakur would be beating him with a stick. And in winters it feels worst on being beaten up. But whatever wound he will get after beating will go away and pain will be momentarily there. But what if he asks him to pay the cost of this missing buffalo; he thought he is a poor man who survives on his daily wages how he will pay back the cost of such an animal. And if he will not be able to pay its cost then he will complain about him to the king, he will be imprisoned in the jail. And he will soil his name as well.

In his heart he prayed to God, 'Oh dear Lord! If you will save me today then I will offer you kheer made out of finest rice I promise you this.' Within few moments Birji reached across Thakur's house. He saw the buffalo which got lost was tied at his door step. To see him there Thakur said loudly, 'Oh Birji today you have not taken my buffalo for grazing.' Within few moments he understood that today he did not bring this buffalo out for grazing, and then how he could have lost it. He thought too much and perhaps winter has frozen his brain completely. He said 'no troubles Thakur Sahib I will take you buffalo for grazing now but today you must get the kheer made and do feed me some because today your buffalo was saved from getting lost.'

Then he told everything about this incidence and told him how grateful he was that buffalo was not lost. And the owner replied while laughing, 'Wow Birji! Whether buffalo has grazed today or not but we will get to eat the Kheer of offering which will be prepared for God.' And both of them enjoyed a meal of kheer in order to celebrate buffalo's return which did not get lost at all.

Moral

Un-necessarily getting panicked is baseless act.

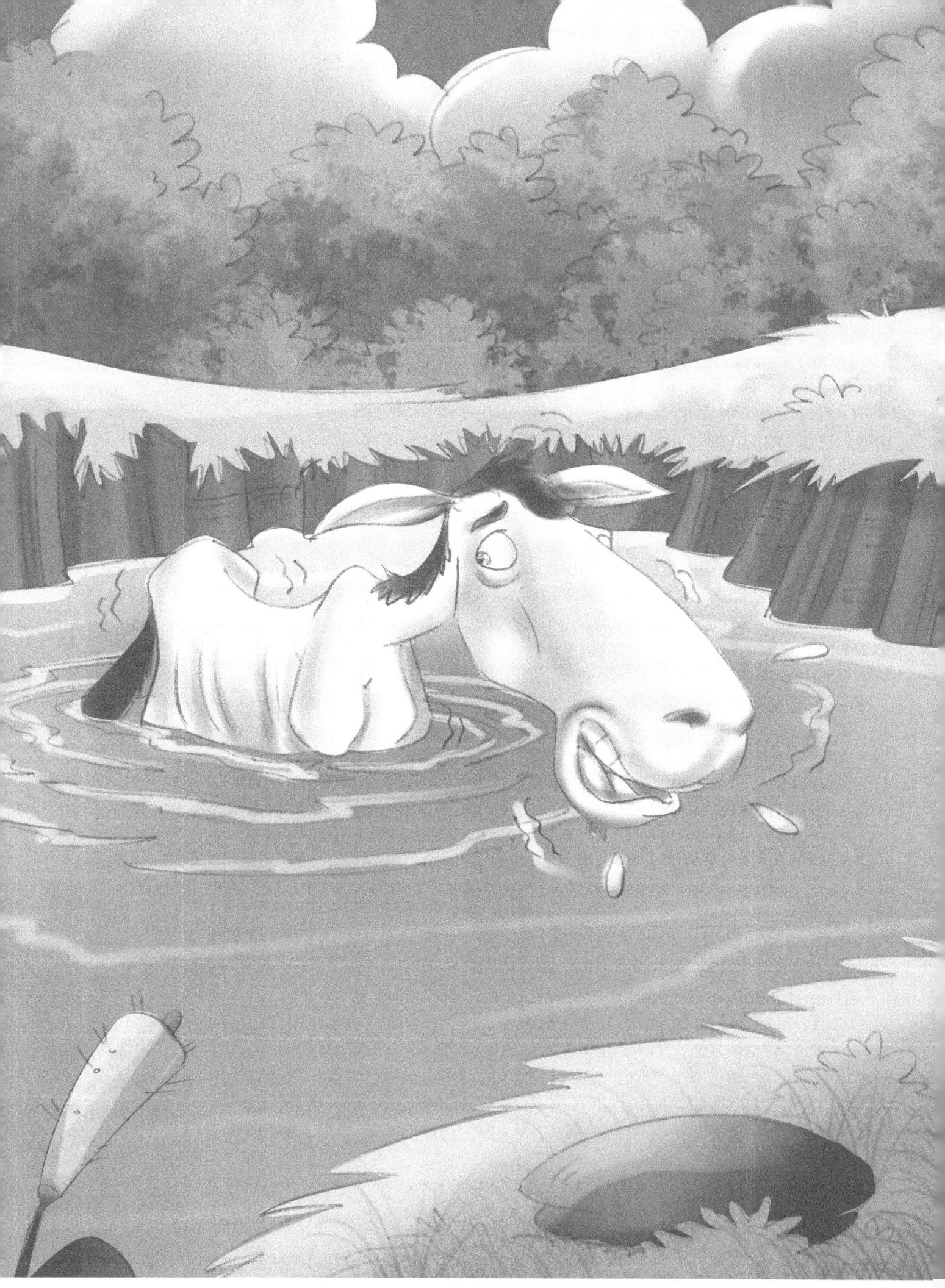

never lose courage

Murli the farmer's donkey fell in a deep ditch. donkey tried to come out of that ditch and struggled a lot, but could not come out. This donkey started to screech in a very loud voice for help. Listening to his cries for help the farmer came running towards that ditch. He felt bad to see his donkey so miserable and helpless he felt bad. He started to think what he must do so that his donkey can come out from this place. After a lot of thinking, the farmer decided to leave the donkey there because he was old now and he was of no use for him. He called all his neighbours and asked them to fill the ditch with mud. And they all started to fill it with mud.

The donkey was horrified to see why all this was happening. He started to hop and jump fast. As soon as they would throw mud on him donkey would jump and shrug the mud off his shoulder. This is how due to the rising level of ground inside the ditch, donkey was able to come out of the ditch. The donkey did not lose his courage till the end. He fought with this ordeal bravely and emerged out of it.

The donkey showed a lot of courage and patience of mind. As soon as people started filling the ditch with earth, he guessed that eventually the ditch will be filled and he would be able to come out of the ditch.

As soon as the donkey came out, he ran way from the place and escaped the bondage of his owner.

He saved himself only due to his presense of mind.

Moral

With presence of mind and courage one can overcome any ordeal.

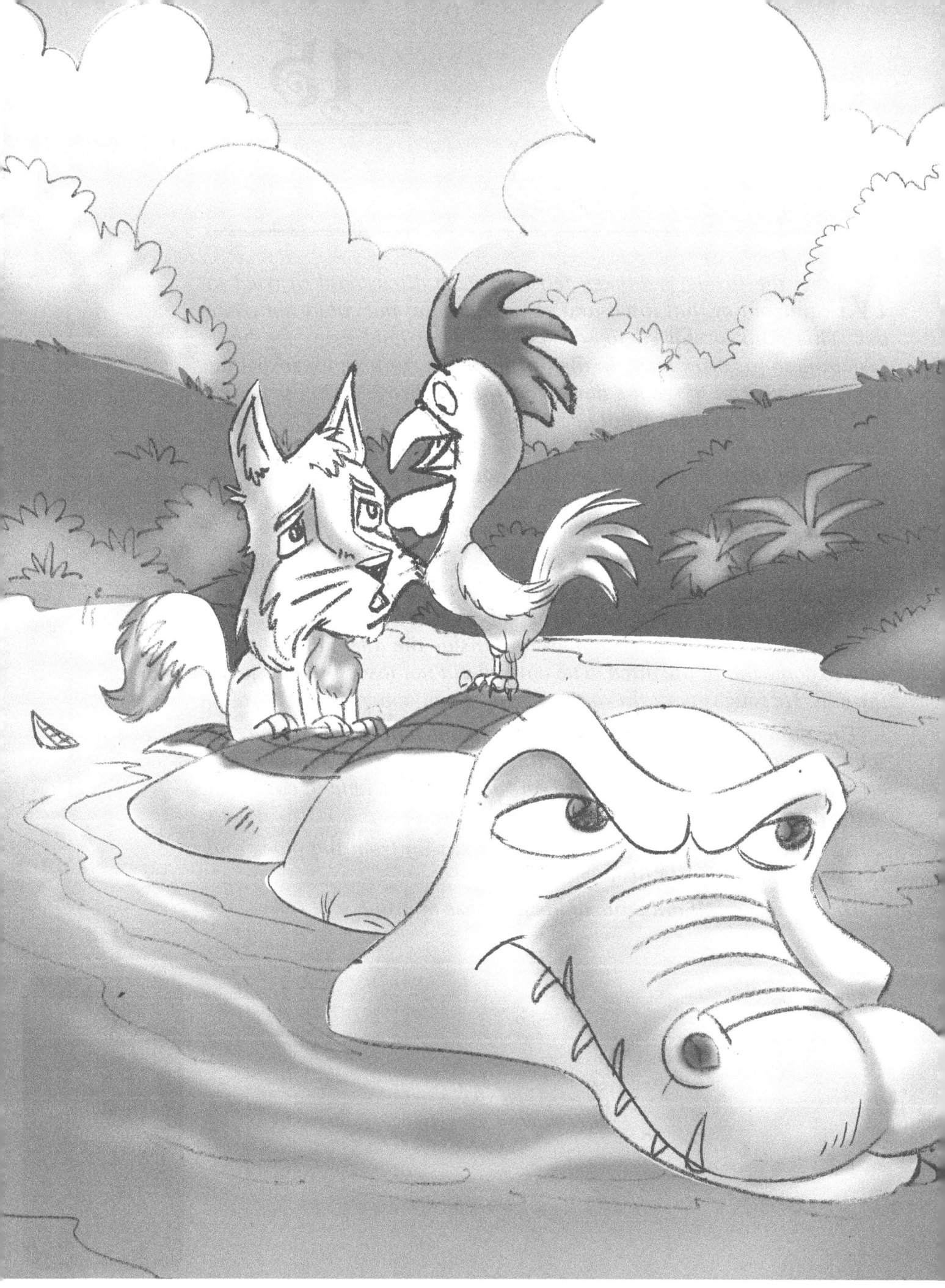

turkey and jackal

*I*n a forest lived a jackal and a turkey. They were good friends. Then one day jackal said to turkey 'you know a good friend is the one who can make his friend laugh, make him cry and when needed save his life. Can you do this for a friend?' Turkey said yes. Suddenly they saw two travellers passing by. One traveller had a huge bundle of wood on his shoulder. Second traveller was carrying his shoes in his hands. Turkey went and sat on the bundle of wood. The traveller walking behind wanted to kill turkey. He threw his shoe towards it, but it flew away. The shoe hit the head of the traveller walking in front. Travellers started to fight. Jackal laughed and said, 'see I have made you laugh but can you make them cry.'

That time a hunter was passing by with his dogs. Turkey said 'now I will show you how I can make you cry. Just go and hide in the hollow trunk of tree in front.' Turkey started to hover on the head of these dogs. Dogs ran after it to catch hold of it. Turkey flew and sat on the same tree where jackal was hiding. Now dogs arrived Hearing his dogs bark the hunter came closer to tree. he got hold of jackal hinding in the tree trunk and dragged him outside. Dogs attacked jackal. Jackal started to cry. Turkey asked, 'did you cry just now?' Jackal replied you have made me cry and laugh as well. Now when you will save my life I will know you are my true friend. We will take the route of the river this time to go to the forest. I have a friend who is a crocodile and he will make us cross the river on his back.'

They met the crocodile and sat on his back. In the middle of the river turkey said in Jackal's ears, 'I think this crocodile wants to eat us.' 'I will fly away but I am worried about you.' Crocodile spoke 'I am feeling very hungry.' Turkey said 'are you thinking to eat my friend?' Crocodile did not say anything and and carried them the bank of river. Then turkey asked jackal 'now do you trust me as your good friend.' Jackal replied, 'yes indeed you saved me but I have to be aware with such a playful friend who can do anything, therefore it would be better if I stay away from such a mischievous friend forever.'

Moral

A friend who is full of mischief cannot be trust worthy. With his work only uncertainty is expected.

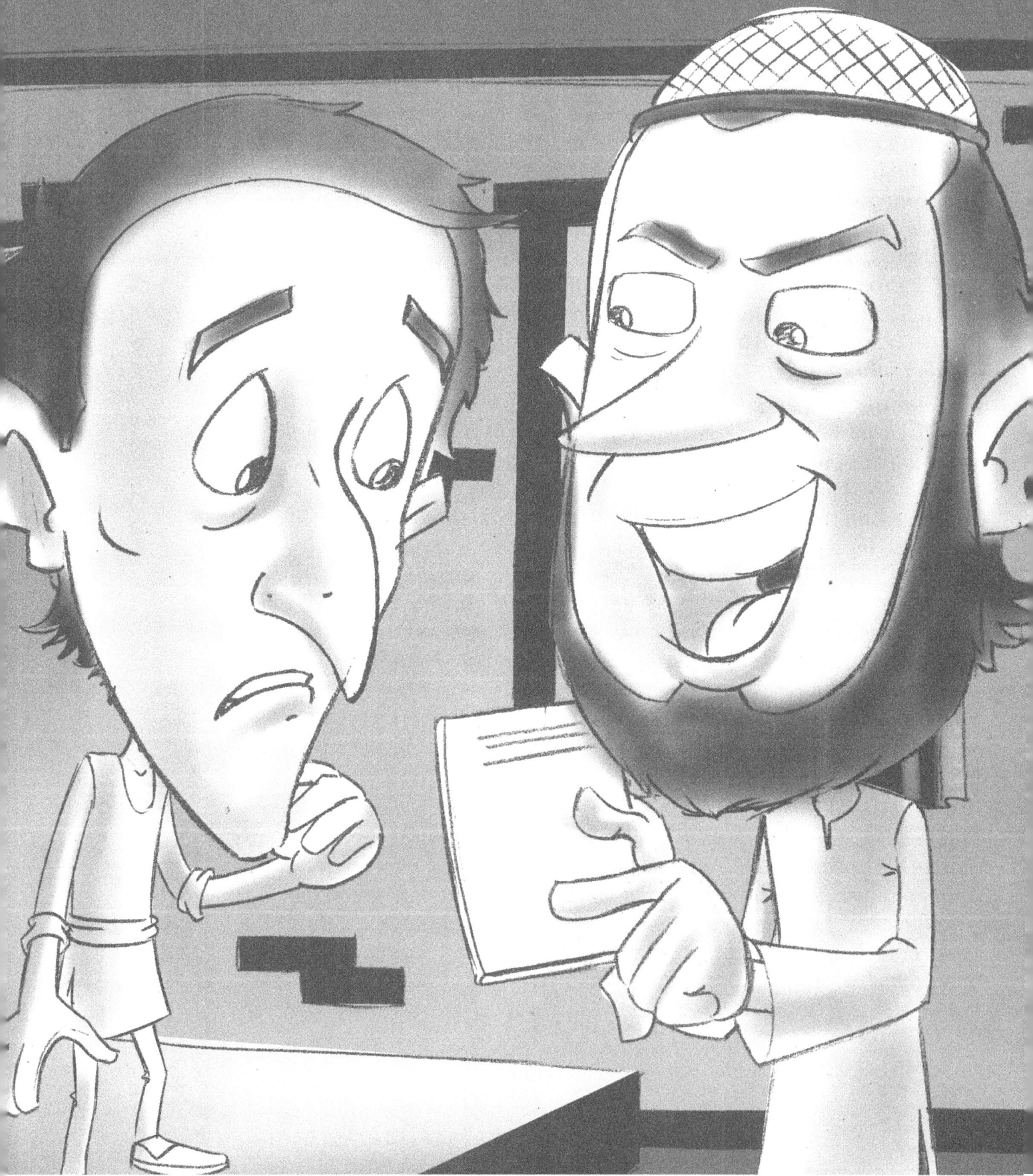

justice of a priest

*O*ne day in the animal fare a priest and Sukhiya a farmer's bulls started fighting with each other. The Priest's bull was stout and strong, that is why he killed Sukhiya's bull in the fight. Sukhiya appealed to priest to give him justice in his court of authority. The Priest read out the definition of law and said, 'if your bull has died fighting with other bull what a priest can do in such matter.' Sukhiya was enraged with this statement. He decided he will take revenge from the priest one day.

Next day Sukhiya bought a new bull. He took care of it for a year. He fed it the best so that it became healthy and powerful. Like every year this year as well village had an animal fare. Sukhiya grabbed an opportunity. He made his bull fight with the bull of the priest. This time Sukhiya's bull was victorious. His bull succeeded in killing priest's bull. As soon as priest learnt about this incidence he summoned Sukhiya to his court immediately. Sukhiya said, 'what can I do in this matter, this all is the result of animals fighting sir.'

But Priest was much cleverer than him. He said, 'the red book says, why the farmer has made both the bulls fight. The farmer raised his bull by feeding him well now he has to bear a fine of hundred rupees with returning the bull in lieu of one which died.' Sukhiya had to pay the fine as well as give a bull in return too. He thought whatever justice a Priest imposes is considered absolute.

Truly, justice is that system of adjusting conflicting interests which makes a group strong and progressive rather than week and retrogressive whereas injustice is a system of adjusting conflicts which make a person weak and retrogressive rather than strong and progressive.

Moral

An influential person says or does is considered right at any cost.

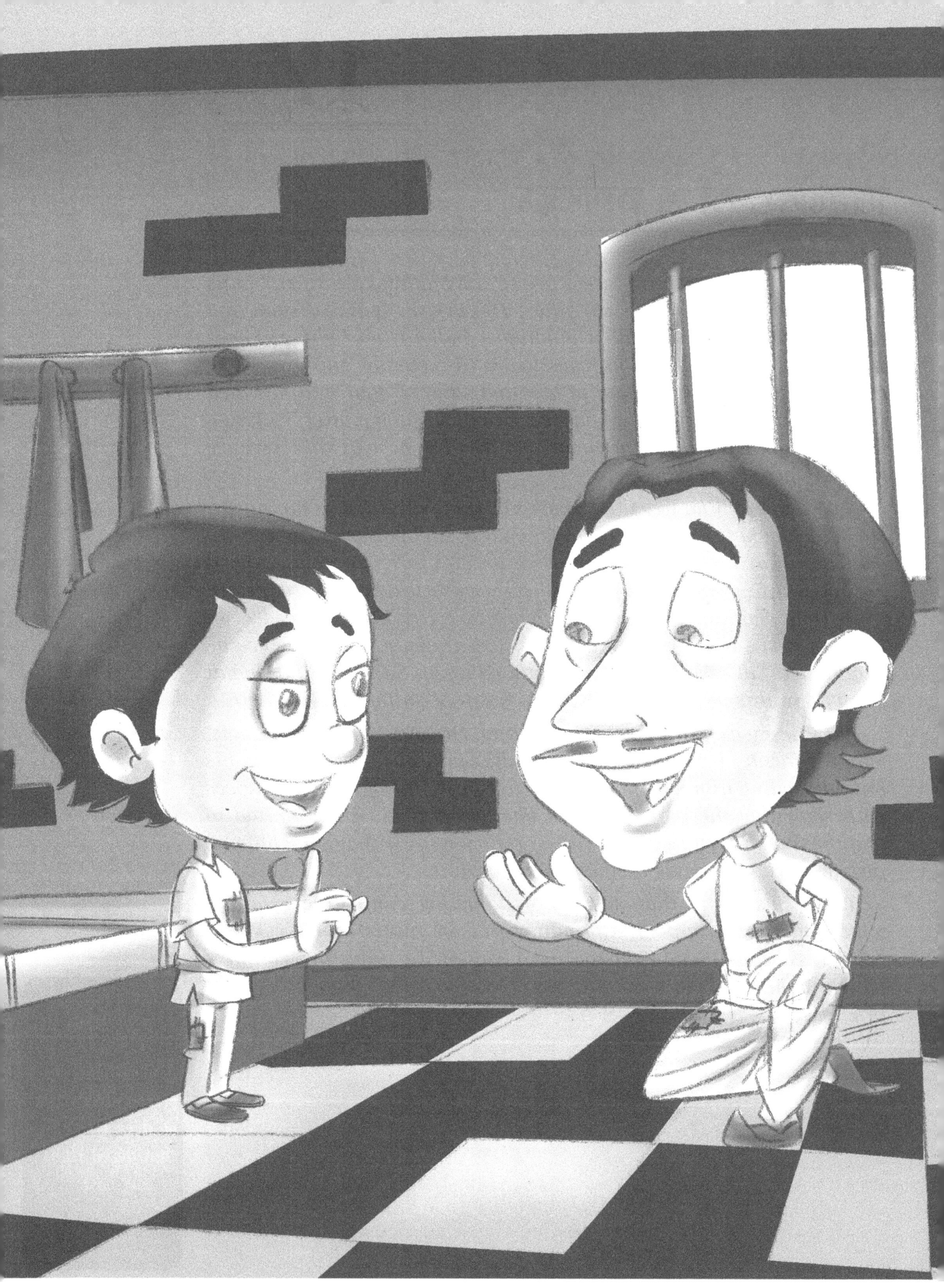

One Penny Elephant

*I*n a village lived a wealthy tradesman. One day he suffered great loss in his business. Within a short time all his saved money was lost. Then one day such misery struck that he had to leave his mansion and had to move in a rented house. He could not get two square meals a day even. One day his son came running to him and said, 'an elephant seller has arrived to do business. Do you remember we used to ride an elephant earlier?'

The tradesman said, 'but our time has changed now.' He added we will have better time someday but for that we have to try working hard'. But his son said that we can still this elephant buy. The elephant seller was ready to sell it to us in one penny. He had struck the deal with him. The tradesman replied, 'we will buy that elephant which is one lakh rupees in cost not the one which is available in one penny. That time we will be able to feed it well. And it will look graceful standing at our doorstep. If we will get it today in one penny then we won't be able to feed it properly. And neither will it look graceful standing at this doorstep.' The son learned two things that day first is any object's demand and usability cannot decide its cost or value.

In fact, there are many things in life that will catch our eye, but only a few will catch your heart.

Grief can take care of itself, but to get the full value and usefulness of a thing, we must have somebody to share the pleasure of value.

Moral

Any such object which we cannot maintain or take care of, we must not keep it with us.

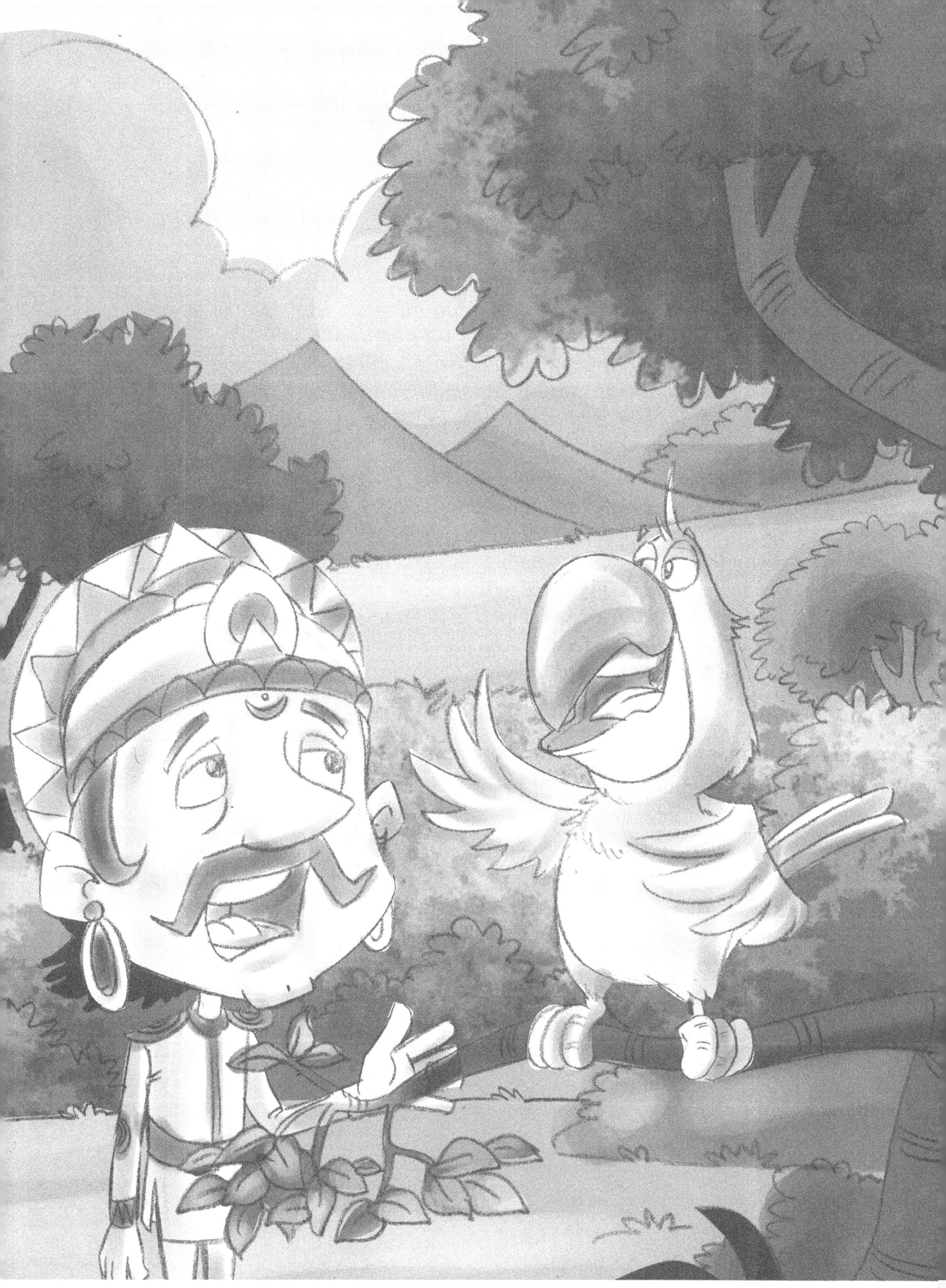

a good company

On a tree lived two parrots. They were real brothers and they looked similar too. One day a storm came. To find a safer place they both flew from the tree. Due to strong wind one of the parrots fell in the camp of thieves and another one fell right in the middle of a hermitage. They had no other place to live so where they fell they started living there.

One day king Chatursen went for a hunting expedition. While looking for a creature to hunt he reached inside the camp of thieves. He was tiered and he sat under a tree to rest. All of a sudden he heard a sharp sound of parrot singing. It was the same parrot which fell years ago in the camp of thieves. It was screaming on top of its lungs, 'here a man is sleeping, who was also wearing gems and jewels worth thousands. Come quick and plunder it.' King understood that he was calling all thieves to arrive there. He immediately sat on his horse and rode it till the end of the jungle and came out of there.

At a distance he saw the hermitage. As soon as he reached inside this hermitage a mellow sound was heard. It was saying, 'King, all hermits were gone to bathe in the river. You may drink water and rest here.' When king saw it was the sound of a parrot. To see him king was amazed. He said, 'few moments away I met a parrot, who was just like you in appearance. His tone was very rude and he was talking about plundering, whereas you are talking with a lot of love. Do you know him?'

'Yes king! it is my real brother. He lives with thieves now and I live here with hermits. This why whatever we hear we repeat the same.' Said the parrot, and now king asked, 'but how you two got separated?' Parrot told everything in detail to the king. When he heard his entire story king said, 'a company's effect always shows on living beings.' This is why one must live in good company.

Moral

A good company or a bad company's effect shows on every one. This is why one must live in a good companionship. It is the wisest thing to do.

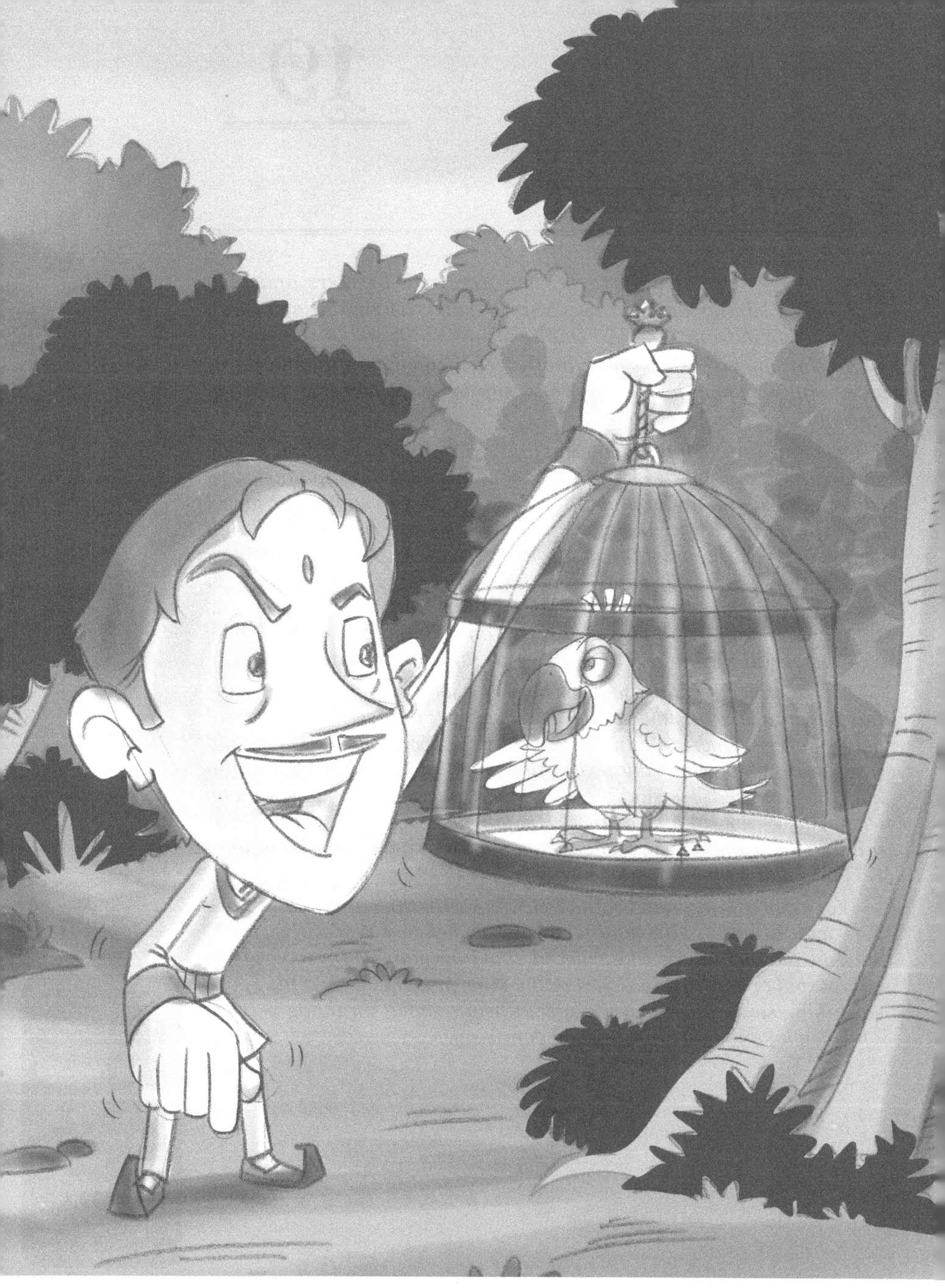

a craming parrot

A person named Manmukh had a pet parrot. He taught the parrot only one word which was 'certainly'. One day he thought why not to sell this parrot to someone. For this act he made a plan. He dug the ground at different places and has put some money in all the ditches. Next day he took his parrot with him and started to tell people 'my parrot is very smart. It can tell me where all money is buried under the ground.'

To hear him say all this villagers started to laugh at him. They said to Mansukh, 'can you prove yourself right?' Mansukh replied, 'why not, see it yourself how my parrot can do such miracles.' He took his parrot along to all those places where he buried his money a night before. He asked his parrot, 'if I will dig here will I find any money here?' parrot replied 'Certainly!' Manmukh started to dig in front of people and dug out the money. In that same crowd there was a youth who was amazed to see parrot's ability and started to think if I will get this parrot then I will become rich instantly. He asked Manmukh 'can you sell me this parrot?' Manmukh felt happy because this is what he desired. But he pretended and said, 'sir, this is my very dear pet. I love my parrot a lot. But if some will make profit through his skill then I will be delighted. I will give you this parrot in lieu of one thousand gold coins.' Then that youth replied, 'but this amount is a lot.' And Manmukh said, 'but you have to give it once, and the parrot will make you earn twice as much.' The youth agreed to Manmukh's offer. He gave him one thousand gold coins and went ahead with his parrot.

After reaching a certain distance the youth stopped. He asked his new parrot, 'if I will dig here will I find money?' parrot replied, 'certainly!' this youth dug up till the end but no wealth was to be found. To listen to his parrot youth kept on digging here or there entire day, but not even a single penny was found. Now he understood that parrot's true owner has cheated him. He was talking to his parrot and said, 'I think I have done a big mistake by purchasing you in one thousand gold coins.' And his parrot replied, 'certainly!' to hear this youth busted out laughing and said, 'first time you have not lied to me. But now I have understood that due to hard work and dedication one can become rich. Not due to some cramming parrot.' To hear all this parrot said again, 'certainly!' then youth said, 'now it is second time that you have not lied. From now on wards you are my pet parrot.' He took his parrot towards his home.

Moral

Before buying anything one must analyse that object thoroughly. Never get pursued by the seller's remarks.

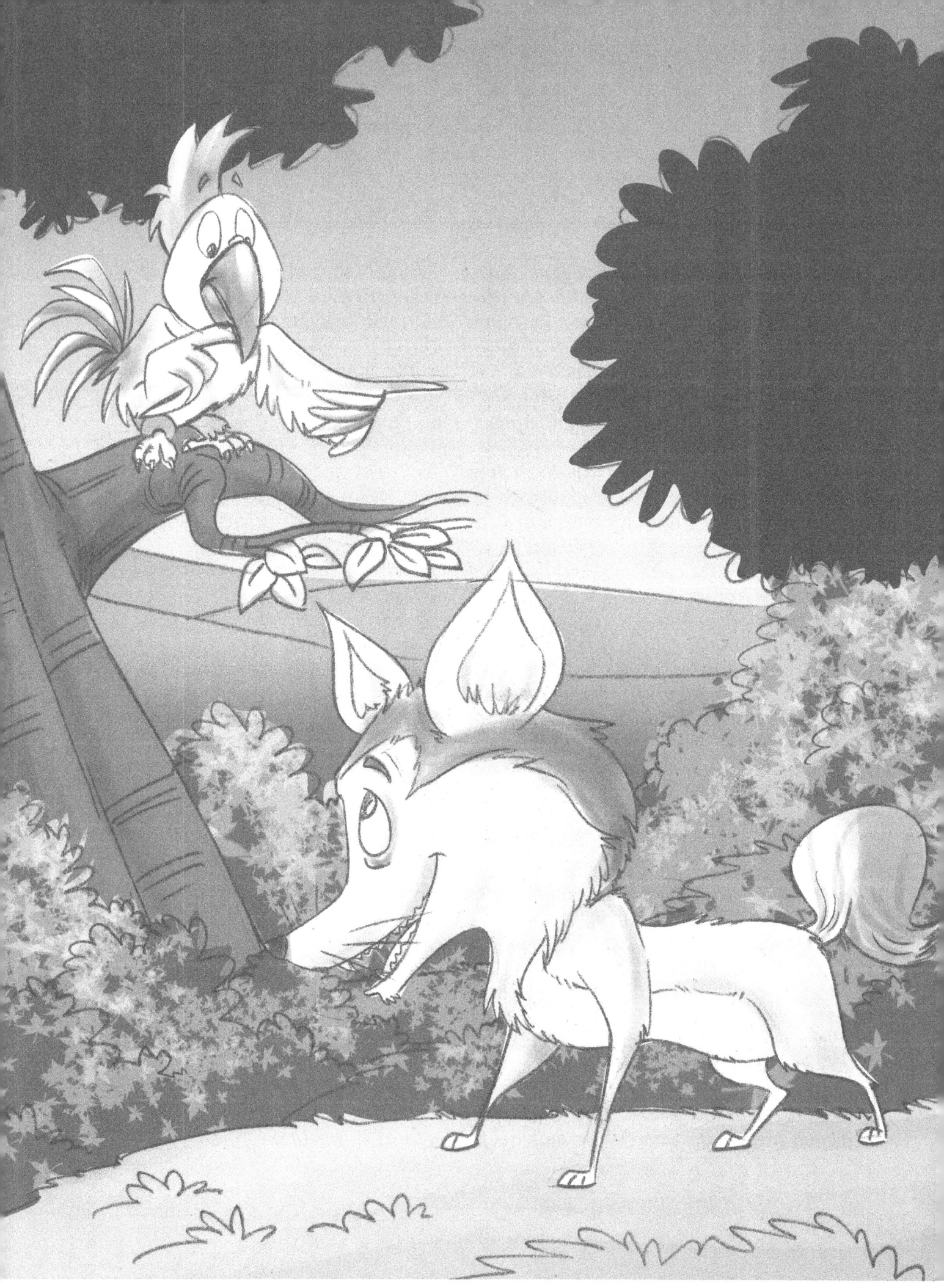

treacherous fox

In a forest lived a treacherous fox. The fox would see a rooster sitting on the branch of a tree every day but she could never catch it to eat. One day fox said to the rooster, 'Oh brother rooster! There is a very happy news for all of us. Just now a message has arrived from the heaven. Which is from now onwards all birds and animals will live together peacefully without killing each other. Now you do not have to be frightened with me anymore, you can come down from the tree. We will sit and talk with each other.'

The rooster replied after listening to her, 'this is indeed a very good news and this is why many of your friends are coming to see me as well.' Fox was amazed to know this and said, 'are those same hunting dogs which keep on looking for foxes to hunt them down.' Rooster said while laughing, 'what happened why you are shivering after knowing about a pack of hunting dogs.' She tried to jump in order to run from there. But then rooster remarked, 'why are you running away from now on wards we all are friends for each other.' Fox replied, 'maybe these hunting dogs do not know about this new rule and by chance what if they feed on me. I will do one thing which is I will meet you later.' To have said this fox ran away from the place. To see her running rooster said, 'never to trust a treacherous mind, they give nothing other than deception.'

Knowledgeable people say that we are more often treacherous through weakness than through calculation. In the similar vein, we can say that wine is a treacherous friend who you must always be on guard against.

Moral

Always stay away from treacherous people; otherwise you will become a part of their fraud.

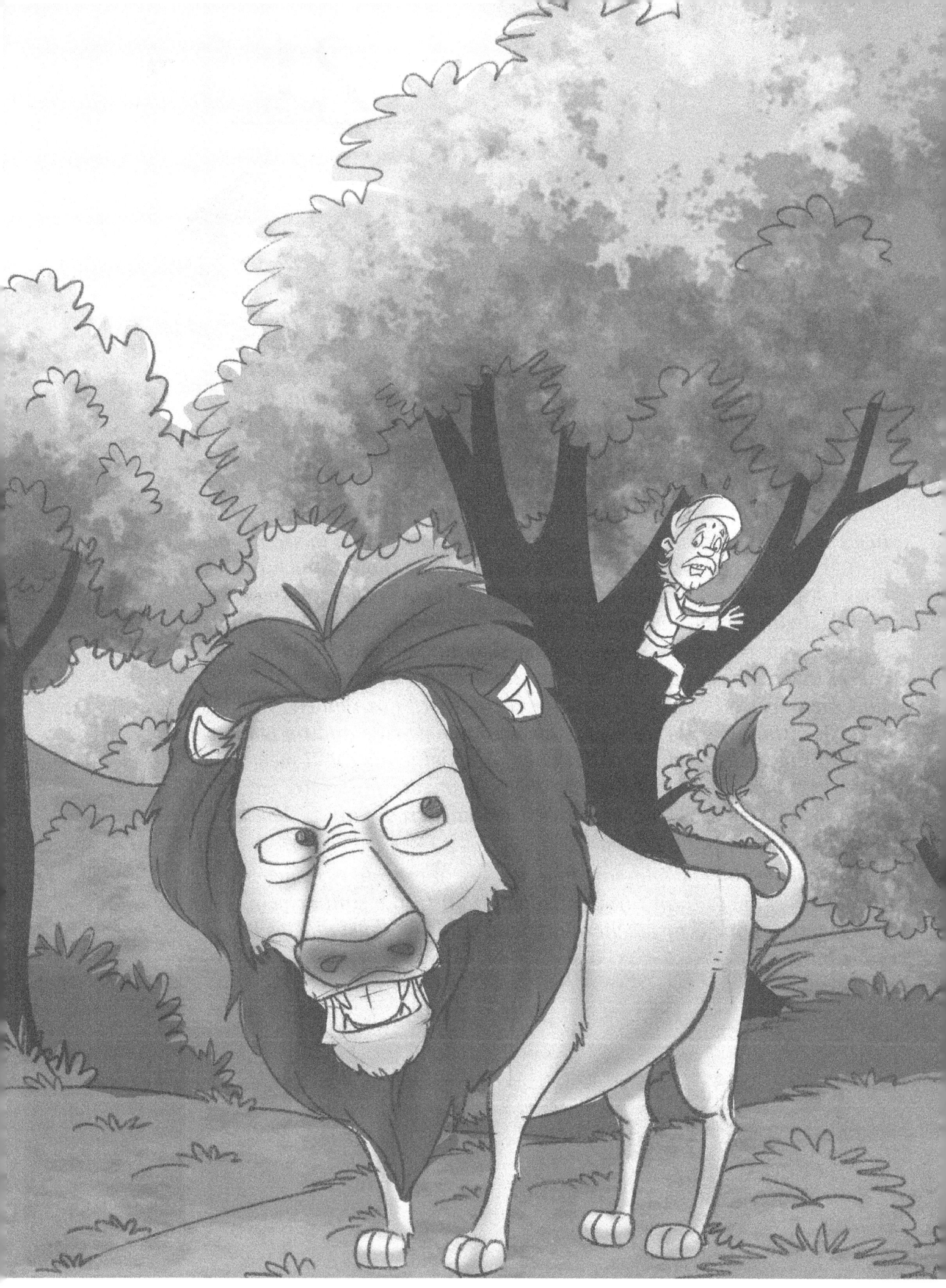

the right use of knowledge

*T*here were five friends. All five of them had no work. But they never desired to work as well. To delay things was their innate habit now. Having fun and sleeping or eating was their entire day's work. To use their brain and body they had almost forgotten. When they received a lot of spiteful comments from their families and society, then they decided they all will learn one skill with its complete knowledge. Four of the friends went in different directions and one of them decided to stay in the village and learn something on his own.

After some time having learnt their knowledge they all met. One of them said, 'I have attained such a knowledge through which I can put back the flesh on a dead beast's body as well.' Second one said, 'I can produce hair and skin back on it.' Third one said 'I can make or re-form all its body parts.' The forth one said, 'I can put life back into it' now the fifth one said, he has learnt the art of climbing trees and chopping wood to earn his living.

To hear fifth one's art of knowing something all four laughed at its ordinariness. To test their knowledge they all went inside the jungle. There they saw a cluster of bones; they lifted them up without knowing whose bones they were. One produced flesh on it; another has put hair and skin back on it. Third one had produced body parts on it and forth one has put life back into it.

Now those bones were of a lion. Lion got alive and ate four of them. And the fifth one climbed a tree and saved himself. This is how in times of need the fifth one's knowledge was proved useful. This is wisely said, if the true knowledge of learning is not known then it is useless.

It is rightly said that words are how people think. When you misuse words or your strength, you diminish your ability to think clearly and truthfully.

Moral

To misuse one's knowledge, can destroy a person's life.

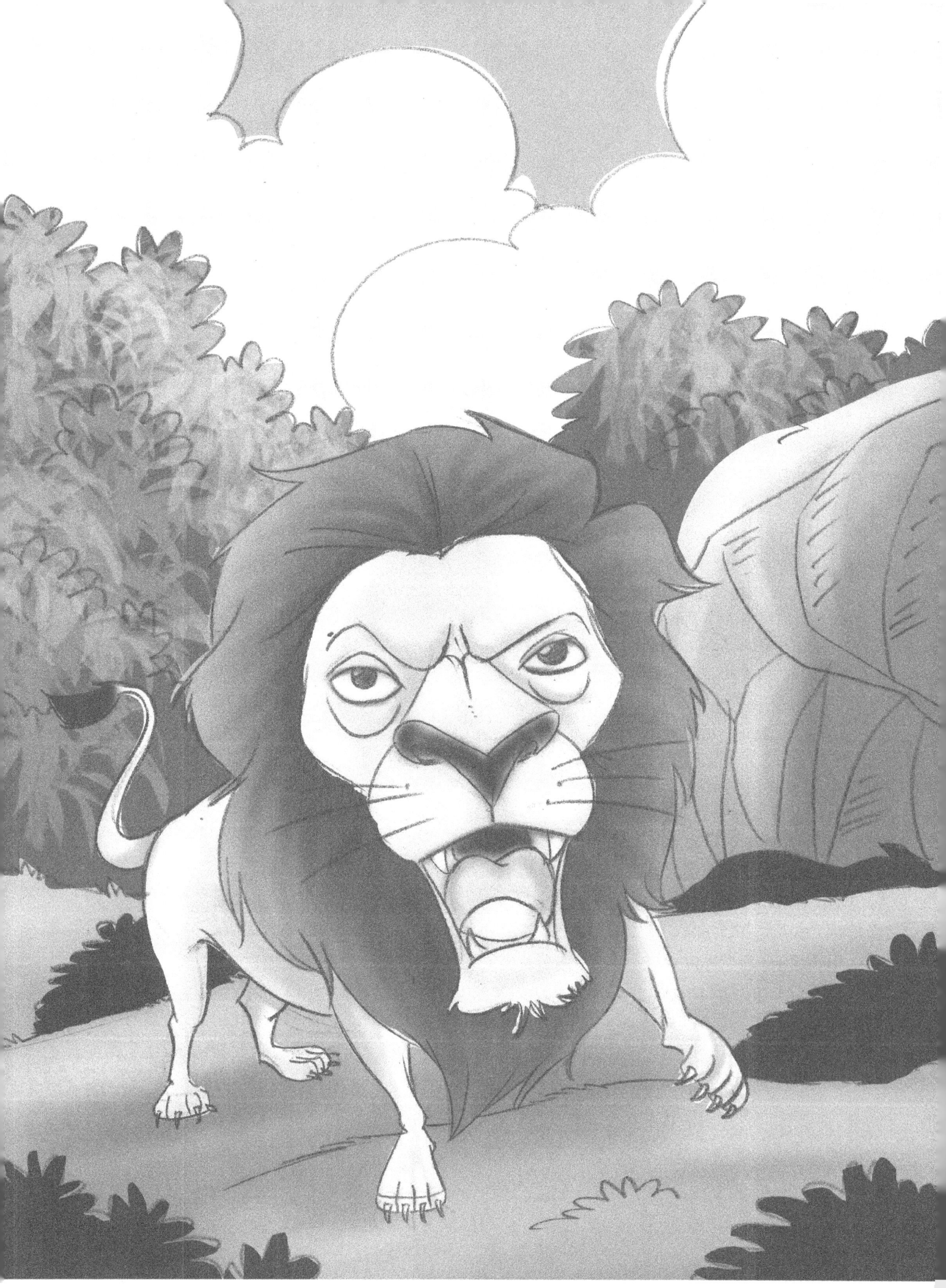

lion's consort

In a jungle these friends used to live, a clever Fox, a shrewd Jackal and a sly Wolf. Three of them thought why not to make friends with the Lion because this is how they can find their prey. Fox took the matter further and said, 'so far we kept on hunting smaller beasts. But if we will be friends with Lion then we can hunt and feed on a bigger animal for days. We will seize the animal and Lion will hunt it down.' All three of them went straight to meet the Lion and explained him everything. And the Lion agreed with their terms and conditions. That same day the Fox, Jackal and Wolf dragged a horned deer which was fat and healthy towards the Lion so that he could kill it. And the Lion killed it in an instance. Now the time came to distribute bounties of their hard work.

Lion said as a wise mediator, 'we are four people therefore we will distribute it in four portions.' They all were very happy to learn this. Lion went close to his prey and said 'first portion would be mine, because I am the king of the jungle, and second portion would be mine as well because I have performed the job of being a mediator. And the third portion would be given to me because one portion already belongs to me. And as far as forth portion is concerned I keep my claw on it and whosoever desire to take it away from me can come and have a fight with me to grab the last share of the hunt.' To hear Lion roar all three saved their lives and went running. All their plans were shattered.

There is a saying that has proven itself time and again that 'A friend should be one in whose understanding and virtue we can equally confide, and whose opinion we can value at once for its justness and its sincerity.'

Moral

Never ever to fall in partnership or consort with a mightier person and never try to show one's cleverness to such a powerful one as well.

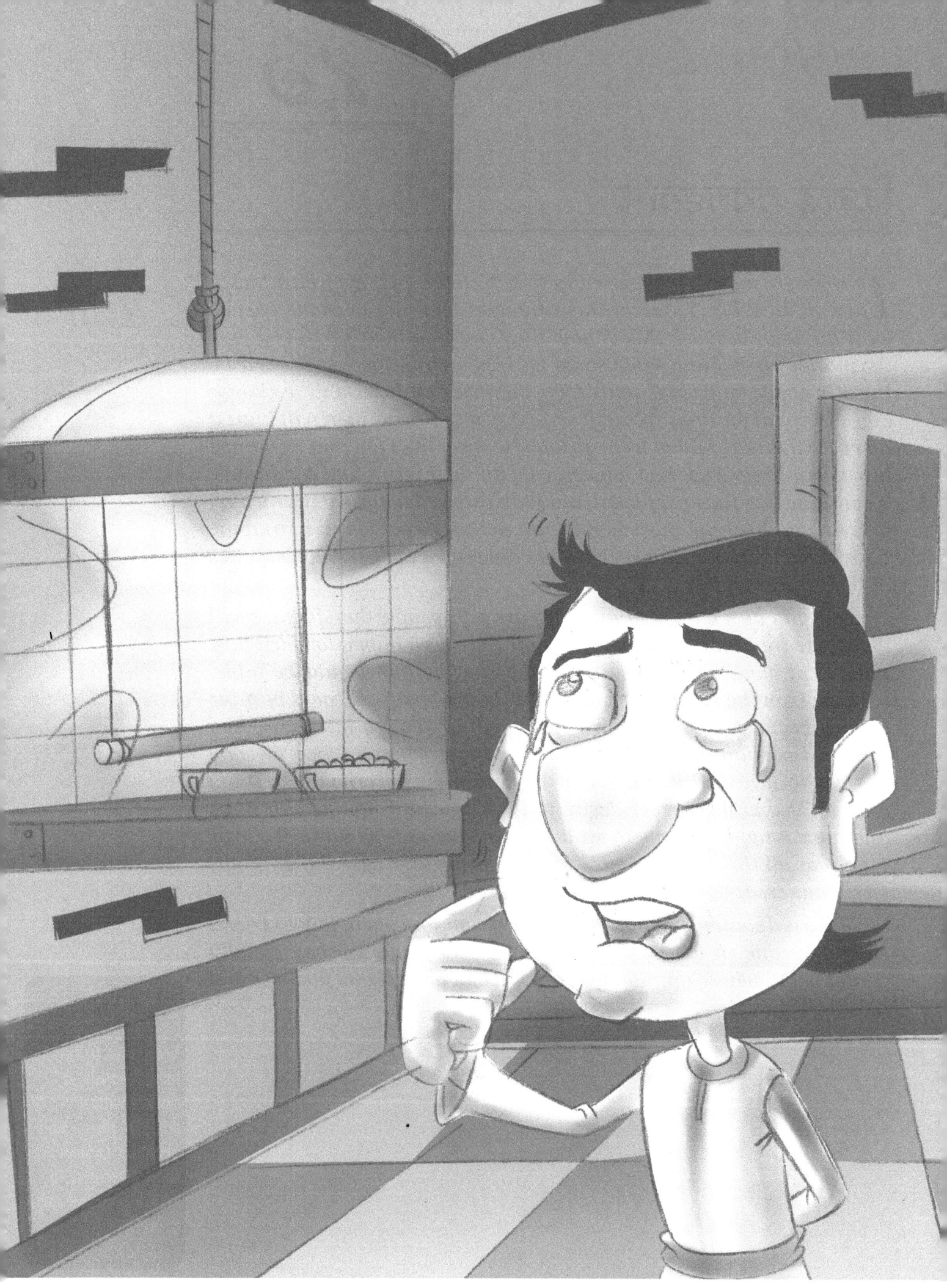

a futile regret

*I*n a village there lived a man called Bhola. He had a very beautiful wife. He always wished to have her in front of him. One day Bhola had to go outside his city for work. There he saw sellers selling beautiful caged birds. Bhola's eyes fell on a parrot who could speak in human language. He bought that parrot. He hung it cage at one corner of his house, but he did not tell his wife that this parrot could speak the human language. After few days he left for some work, and when he returned back after a long time he asked his parrot 'tell me what all happened here in my absence?'

The parrot said, 'your wife does not show a moral behaviour.' After listening to what this parrot told him the man scolded his wife and locked her in the house. The wife wondered how did her husband got to know about her behaviour? The wife asked every maid in her house but all of them refused doing so. She thought it is the work of this parrot. She plotted to prove how this parrot wrong. One day when Bhola left for work, his wife told her maids, 'one of the maid will work on the flour mill tonight so that parrot must think the clouds are roaring outside. Another maid will sprinkle water on the parrot in such a fashion that he thinks it is raining.'

When Bhola returned home he asked his parrot to report about the previous night to him. Parrot replied, 'throughout the night the clouds were roaring and I got drenched in the rain.' After listening to this the man was perplexed. He thought that not even a single drop of water fell last night and this parrot thinks it rained heavily.

He concluded that whatever he told me about my wife was complete lie. In anger he killed his parrot and started trusting his wife again. But this trust did not last long. Soon enough his neighbours started complaining about his wife in the same fashion, as the parrot. After learning the truth Bhola was remorseful about his killing the parrot. He could do nothing other than regretting what had already happened.

Moral

After committing the mistake it is futile to keep on regretting it.

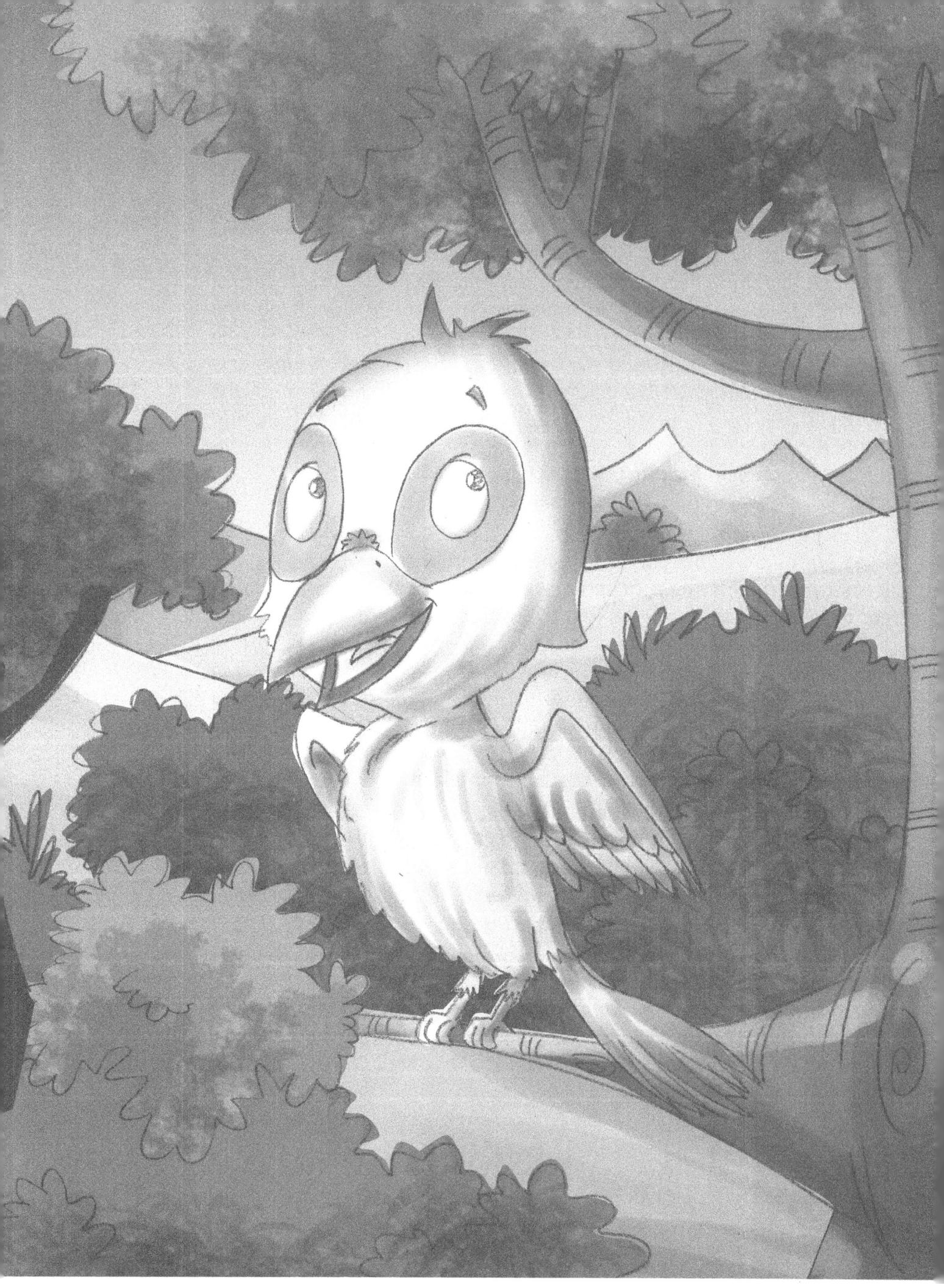

a talkative bird

One day a bird found a pearl. The bird made a nest right outside the king's palace on the tallest tree, and started singing- 'I am richer than the king.' When king heard this he grew very angry. King asked his soldiers to find whatever the bird had in her nest and to take it away from her. The king's soldier went to her nest and took away the pearl from her and brought it back to the king.

In evening when the bird returned she got to know that king's soldier came and took away her valuable pearl. The bird started screaming 'oh the king is so poor he stole my pearl from me.' When king got to know this he asked his men to keep the pearl back in her nest. When this happened this bird started singing again-'king is scared of me that is why he has returned my pearl back to me.' This time king ordered to imprison the bird. Even after getting caged the bird did not stop singing- 'King is my servant and this cage is my home now.' now king got furious and decided to kill this bird.

His minister tried to stop the king by saying, 'this bird is talkative. And talkative people go on taking without acknowledging time and place. And to mind what they say is foolishness and no point to stick it to one's heart.' After listening to this king agreed and freed this bird out of the cage. While flying away the bird could not help her habit and spoke again- 'I have defeated the king.' But this time no one paid any attention to her.

It is said talkative people say so many thing out of habit. They don't actually mean what they say. Hence one should not pay much attention to the words of talkative people. They need not be taken seriously.

Moral

The one who talks the most, nobody should pay any heed to what he says.

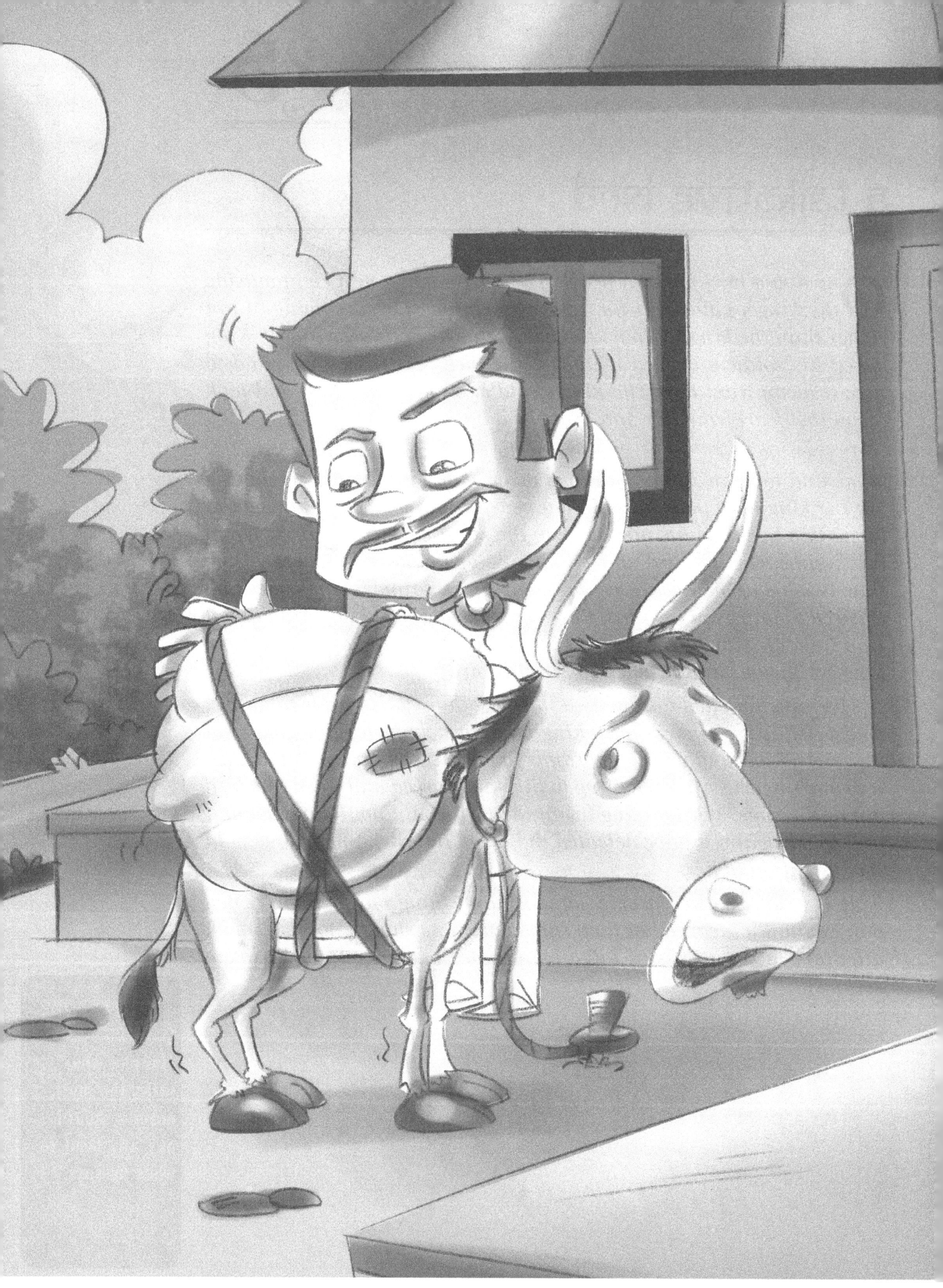

26

doing of an evil master

*L*ong-long time ago a man named 'Bilas' lived in Hastinapur and he was known to be a miser. He had a mule. He would take a lot of work from that poor animal, but would never feed this mule proper food. Day and night mule would work and due to lack of good food mule was getting weaker and weaker. Even then Bilas would take a lot of work from it. One day seeing mule's poor health Bilas thought what if it dies someday then what he will do without it? So he decided to come up with some sort of idea that he must arrange for his fodder's expense to take work out of it and to do something so that he has no need to pay for its food as well.

One day Bilas brought the hide of a dead tiger. He would make his mule wear this tiger's skin. And he would leave it in other's field to graze. Field guards would see the mule and run away from there thinking it was a tiger roaming in their fields. And the mule would graze freely in those fields. To have received a good diet in few days mule got his strength back. Then one day the owner of the field thought that why his crop is always eaten and from where this tiger has started to come here? And this tiger never used to come here. Then he plotted a scheme to kill this tiger.

He wrapped himself in a black coloured blanket and placed himself in the same field at a safer distance. When this mule saw this fellow sitting he thought it is a mule just like him. And due to its nature it started screaming in its mule voice towards the other fellow mule. Then it was simple for the owner to understand what the matter was. It was a mule wearing a tiger's skin. He jumped over that mule and started beating it so much that it fell unconscious. It is said wisely that one must remain away from the services of a bad owner or employee.

It is said that no matter how much you try to coat your personality one false action or the other will reveal your true self. It is always advisable to remain what you ore and not copy someone with an intent to cheat.

Be yourself. This is the true moral of this short story.

Moral

To wear a tiger's skin cannot make the other a tiger, it's essential nature will always remain the same.

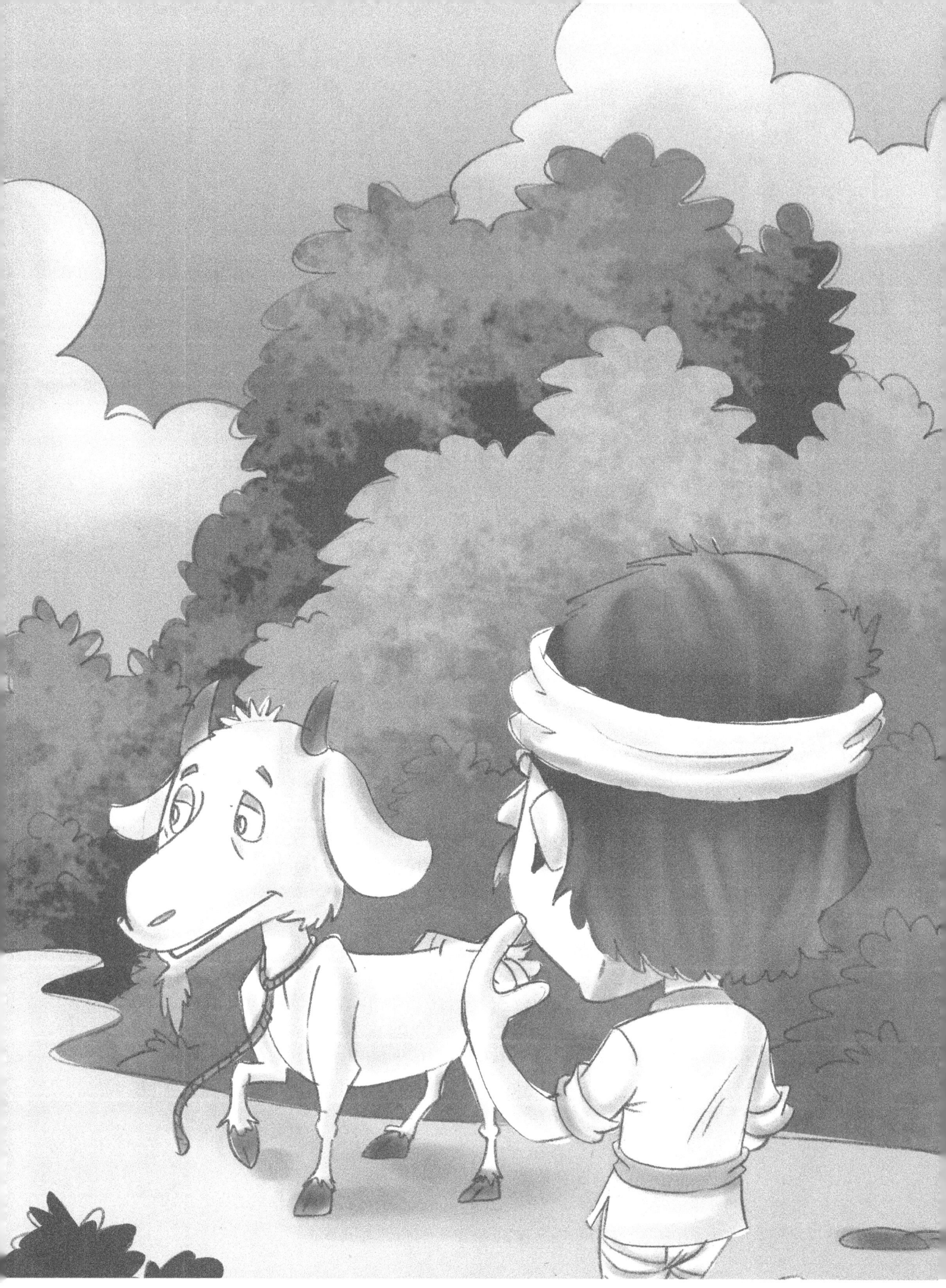

the robbers plot

Once a man called Ramashankar was going someplace while keeping a goat on his shoulders. Three robbers saw him and decided to steal his goat. All three of them plotted against him. All three of them stood at three different points a mile away from each other. As soon as Ramashankar crossed the first thief with the goat on his shoulder, the thief said, 'oh pedestrian! From where are you coming?' Ramashankar replied 'I am coming from a nearby village oh brother.' Then the thief spoke again, 'that is alright but why are you carrying this dog on your shoulder? Is it sick?'

Ramashankar said 'you find this goat as a dog, what a fool you are.' The thief replied, 'alright if you consider this dog a goat it is fine with me.' Ramashankar ignored this man and went ahead. He went a little ahead and then he found out another thief and he also told him that his goat is actually a dog. Ramashankar called him a fool and went further.

After reaching a certain distance he thought whether he is into some kind of delusion? Two people said the same thing to him. He has put his goat back on the ground and started and looked at it from every angle. When he got convinced that it is a goat then very happily he has lifted it on his shoulder again and started walking ahead but now his mind was not stable on this matter. After a while third thief appeared. He also deluded Ramashankar after telling him that it is a dog not a goat.

Once again he has put his goat on the ground and checked it thoroughly. When he got convinced that it is a goat not a dog he started to walk ahead. It is believed that if you speak a lie again and again in convincing fashion then it will appear as truth. Something similar happened with Ramashankar. He was made to believe that it was not a goat but a dog. His own sensibility was put under question. When this thought came in his mind again he dropped that goat then and there and went back to his home. This is what these three thieves wanted they took the goat and sold it in a nearby village.

Moral

Trust one's own brain, and never get persuaded by others.

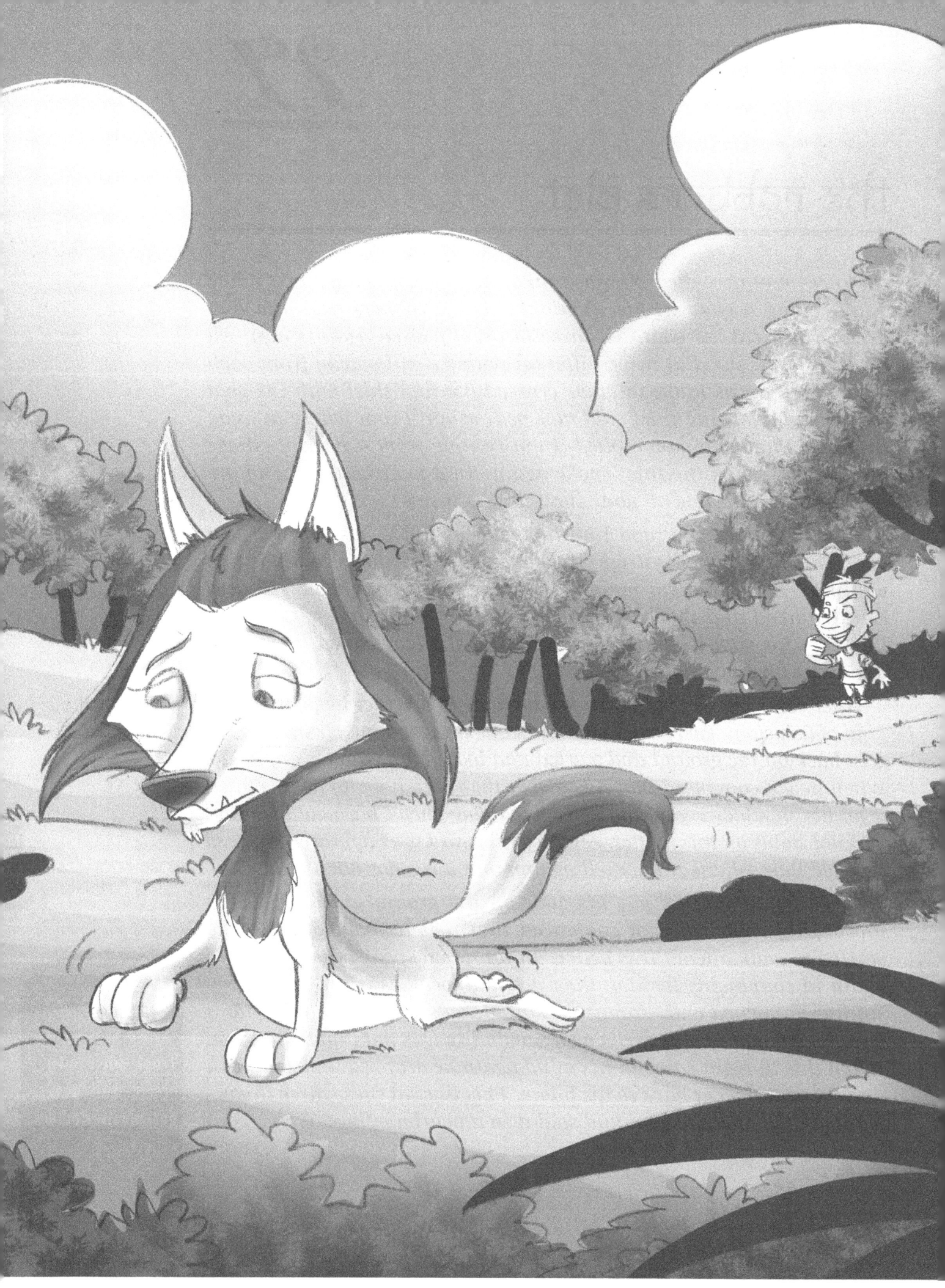

hard work

In a forest lived a Fox. Her frontal legs have gone bad. Right next to the forest a village was located, where a person called Mangoo lived. Whenever he saw that fox he would think it's both legs are crocked, then how she manages to gather food for himself. To solve this mystery Mangoo decided to follow this fox one day and he went straight to the forest. He saw one lion was feeding on an animal. Whatever lion wanted to eat he ate as much as he wanted and left the remaining portion of food for the fox. Mangoo thought this fox cannot hunt her own food that is why God has sent food for her through the medium of lion. He thought when God takes care of all his creation then I must spend my life comfortably and he will provide me food. God will take care of me. From next day onwards Mangoo left all his work and sat at home resting.

He wowed, till God sends food for him he will not eat a single morsel of food at all. In this desire he spent a lot of days without eating. His body grew very weak. His strength to work has also depleted but no food from God arrived. One day he made complains to God.

God replied, 'when you were working then I made sure I will be sending you your daily morsel. But now you have gone astray. And you are comparing yourself with a disabled creature. You were always in a god condition. With your foolishness you have made your body grow so weak that you cannot work now. If I will keep on giving food to everyone then no one will work in this world. To work hard and earn is the duty of every human being and you have forgotten it.'

To hear God say these things Mangoo realised his mistake. He asked for forgiveness to God. By now he understood that God helps everyone. A person who runs away from hard work even God doesn't help him.

Moral

God does not help lethargic and foolish people, those people who work hard get God's bounties.

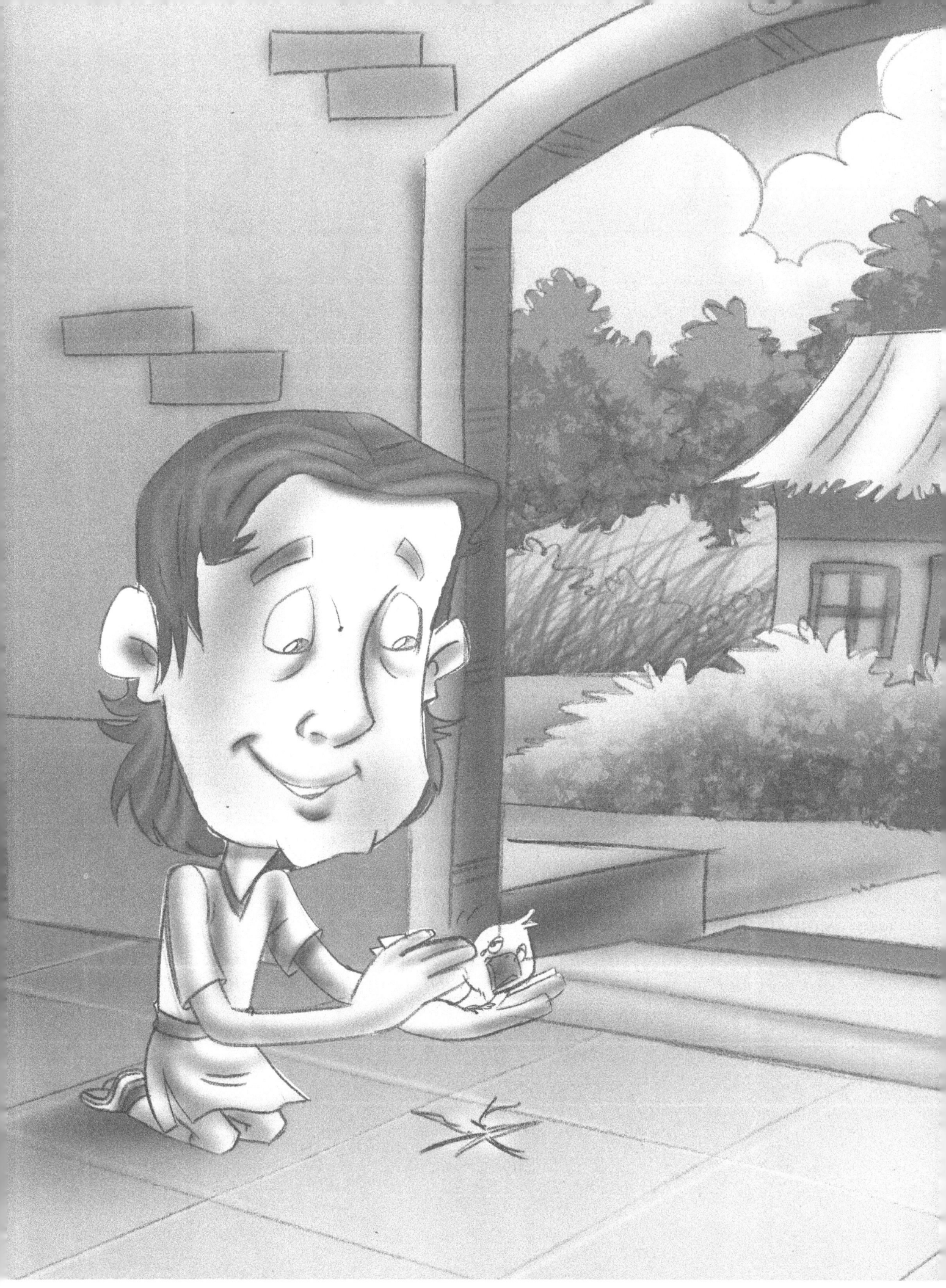

the good and the bad

Right outside Sohan's house a bird made its nest. And laid eggs. And one day eggs hatched as well. Once the male and female birds were not around a small baby bird fell from the nest and broke one of its legs. Sohan picked up that fallen bird and put medicine on its broken leg and placed it back in its nest. When this baby bird grew up and started to fly, it came flying one day and placed one grain of rice on Sohan's palm. Sohan buried that grain in this front yard and forgot about it. One day woke up and was surprised to see at the place where he has buried that grain of rice, a lot of diamonds and gems were glistening on the soil.

Now he understood why the bird was trying to pay back his favour. With a naïve heart he narrated the entire story to his neighbour Mohan. Mohan also felt happy because a bird has also made a nest at his doorstep and it contained a lot of small baby birds. He went straight to his house. And he fetched out one small baby bird from the nest and threw in on the ground. But still it did not break its leg. So he broke its one leg and tied a bandage around it and made it sit again in its nest. When the bird grew up it came flying with a grain of rice and gave it to Mohan. Mohan sowed that grain in his front yard and kept on waiting for it to become agem yielding plant. At the place where he has planted that grain Yam Raj came out of that seed and dragged Mohan with him to Yamnagri.

It is true that the biggest men and women with the biggest ideas can be shot down by the small lest men and women with smallest minds. You possess a potent force that you either use for good or bad, hundreds of times. You harvest what you sow.

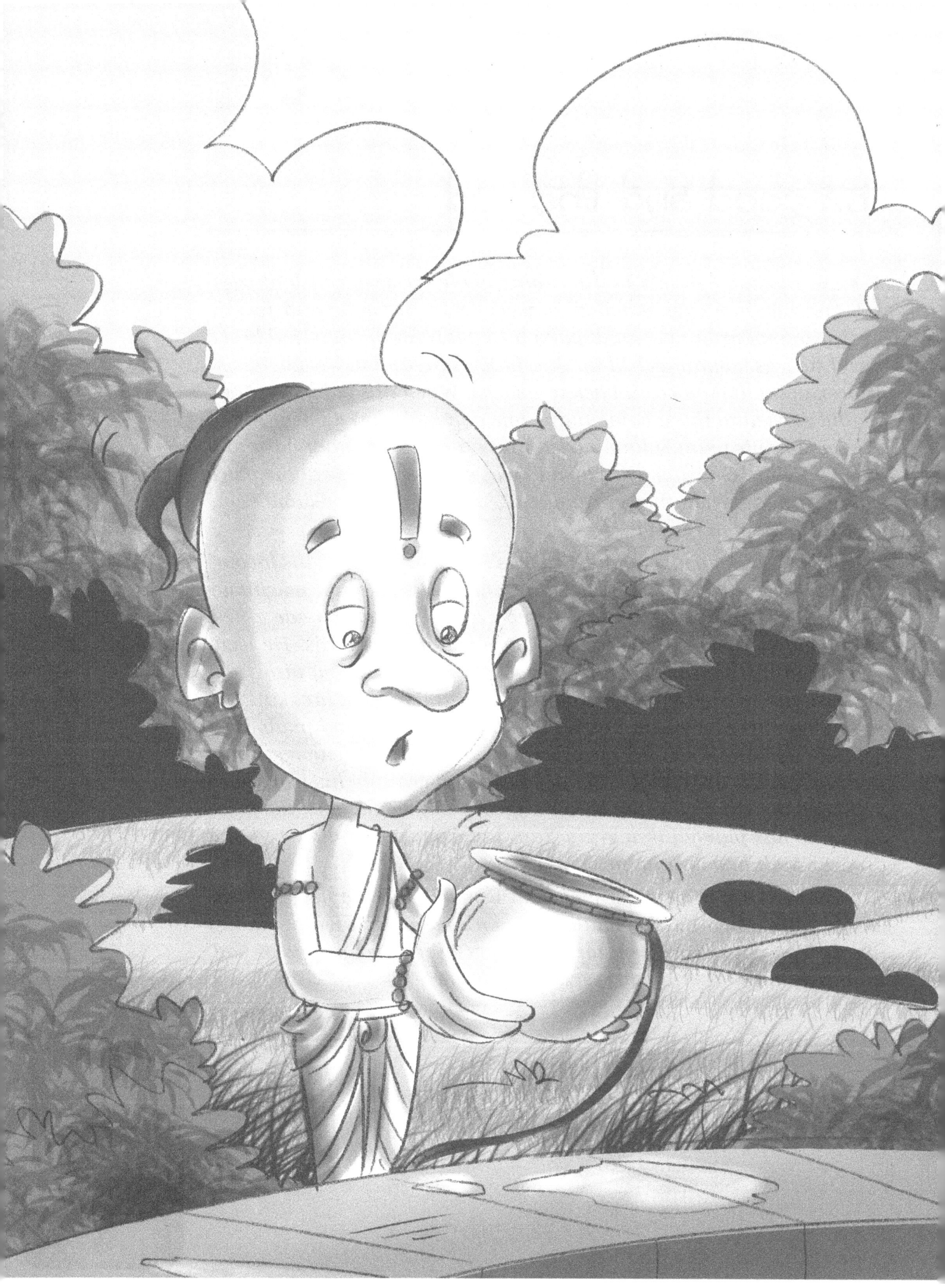

a valuable lesson

There was a saint. He believed whatever a human being needs God gives it to him. His belief was so firm on God that whatever he could ask for God immediately granted to him. Therefore, he would never hold on to anything close to him. The saint use to travel a lot therefore he will always keep a small cask and a rope to draw water to quench his thirst. Once he was on his way and he felt very thirsty, but nearby he could not find any source of water. He walked a bit more but he was extremely thirsty by now. After walking a long distance he saw there was a well, which was full of cold water. And a deer was drinking water from it.

When the deer was done with drinking water from this well he immediately reached towards it. But strangely he sees the water level of this well has sunk very low. The saint was horrified to look at it. He had seen from his own eyes that this well was full of water till the upper level and that deer was drinking water from it comfortably. How it it became so his mind cannot understand this. Now his thirst has almost vanished. He stood up and started thinking what the cause of it was. Only then a voice emerged from this deep well, 'why are you getting startled? The deer did not have a rope or a cask with him; therefore I made water approach towards the deer's mouth. But you are equipped with a rope and a cask both that is why water level went down. You may drink water on your own.'

The saint threw his rope and cask away started walking ahead of that place without having his thirst quenched. All of a sudden a voice was heard again, 'where are you going? I was just testing your patience. You may go and drink the water.' Saint drank that water with a lot of love and when he walked away from that place he left with a very valuable lesson, that one must trust God but also one must work accordingly.

Moral

God helps those, who help themselves.

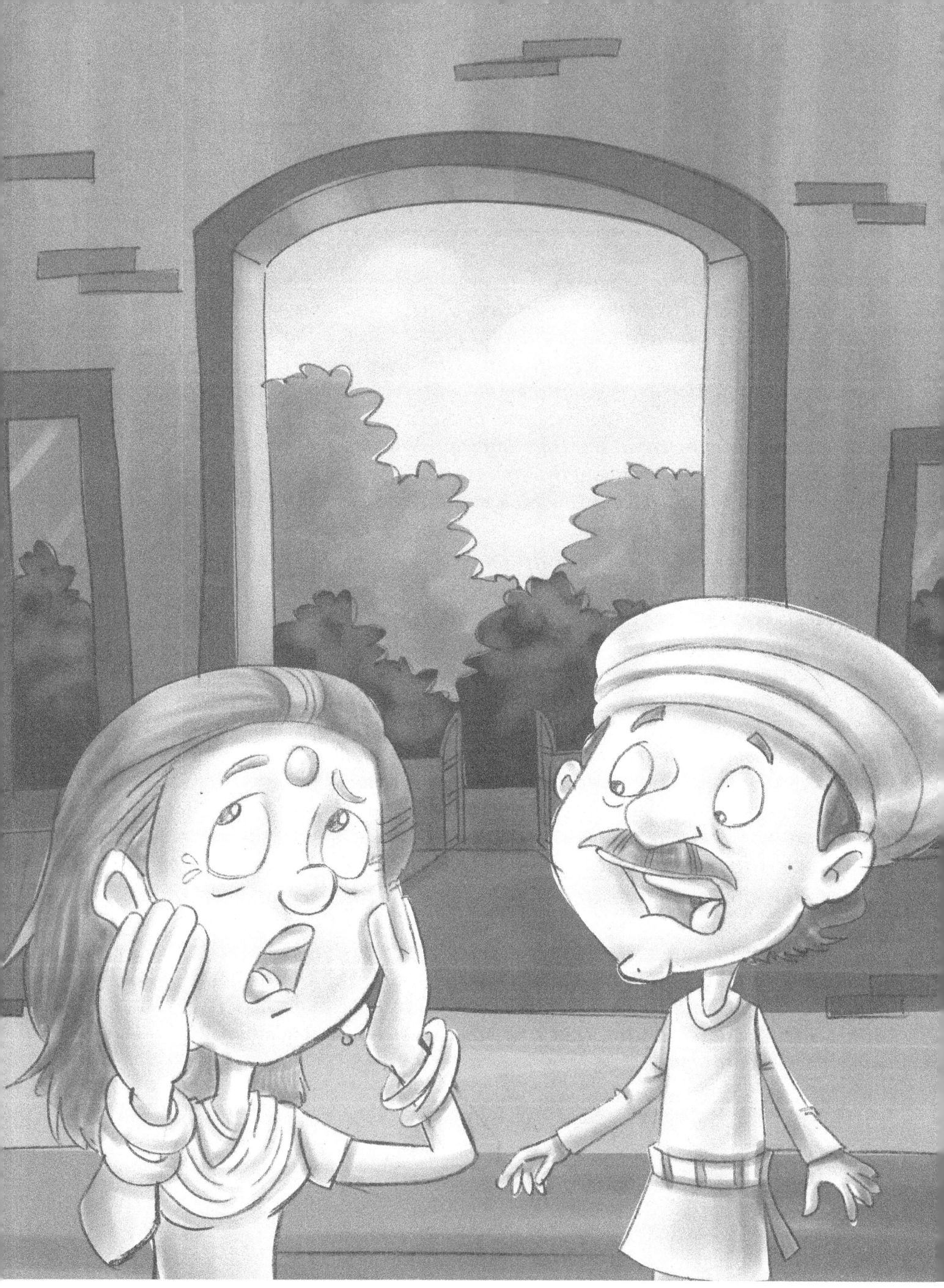

31

Cleverness of the daughter in law

In a village there used to live a man called Radhe. His work was to make toys out of mud. His only desire was get his son married in a nice and well off manner. In the marriage procession his son must come on the back of an elephant. But there was no elephant in his village. When the time of his son's wedding arrived all the arrangements were made but they were worried from where to get an elephant now. Someone told him in the neighbouring village there is a man called Hastimal Seth, who had an elephant at his place; if he will agree to give his elephant then this matter will be resolved. Radhe persuaded Hastimal to give his elephant for the wedding procession. Radhe's son was riding the elephant and went ahead to get his bride on its back. But bad luck took over the poor elephant's life and the elephant fainted, it later died on the spot.

Once the marriage got over and then came the time to return the elephant, Radhe decided to tell Hastimal about this mishap that it will not be possible to return his elephant now, he and his son will return every penny as the worth of that elephant. But Hastimal was strong on his will. He wanted the same elephant which he had given. Radhe tried to persude him a lot but he did not budge and he threatened him that this matter will get resolved in the king's court. When distressed Radhe reached home then his new daughter in law heard everything in detail and said kindly bring Hastimal Ji to our home and will return his elephant to him.

Before Hastimal arrived the new daughter in law shut the door of the house and on the other side of the door she piled all earthen toys one by one onto each other. As soon as Hastimal arrived he tried to knock open the door. And one by one all toys fell and got broken. And she started crying,' oh! You have broken all my earthen toys and vessels'. Seth Hastimal replied 'why worrying so much for earthen toys, take money in lieu of them'. Then the daughter in law said 'but I want the same earthen toys and vessels just like you want the same elephant.' Seth Hastimal realised everything time. He said to the daughter in law, 'you are right dear daughter whether it is an elephant or earthen toys and vessels, everything will become one with this mud someday.'

> **Moral**
>
> Cleverness can mend anything even in worst situations.

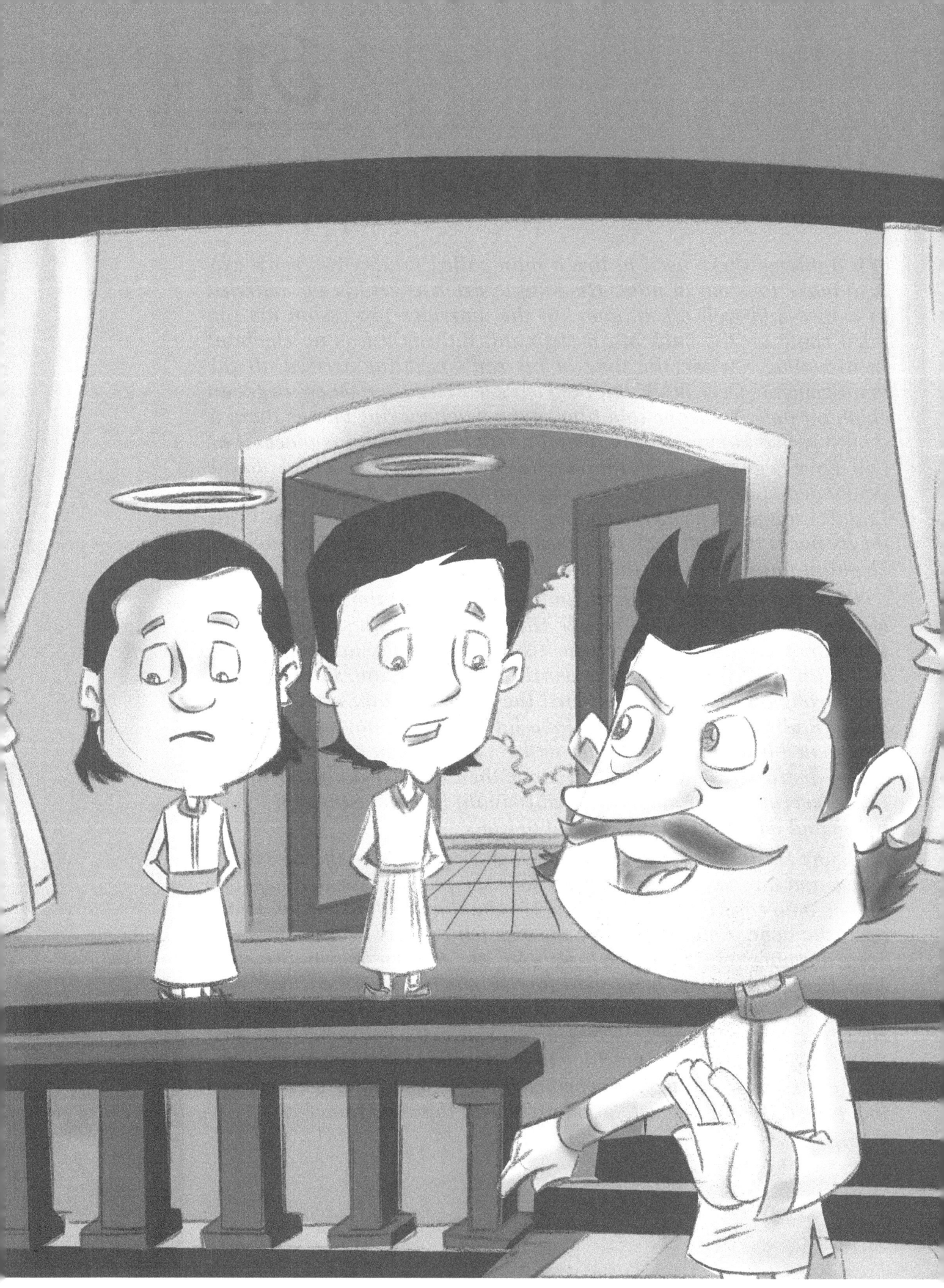

two angels

Two angels were roaming around this world. They decided to spend their night at an extremely rich and greedy trader's house. When they went inside that trader's house he did not treat or welcomed his guests properly. He said, 'if you two desire to spend a night here, then go and sleep in the basement right below my storage room.' They both went into the basement to spend their night. When they were spreading their bedding on the floor they noticed a hole in the wall. When they saw what lies on the other side of the wall they saw a room full of gold coins. One of the angels sealed that hole immediately. Another angel saw him doing so but he remained quiet.

Next day they went to live with a poor farmer. Farmer and his wife welcomed them very warmly. Whatever they had to eat in their house they fed that to those angels. They gave their own beds to them to sleep and they themselves slept on the floor. In the morning when they got up they saw how both farmer and his wife were sitting and crying. They got to know the only source of their income was a goat which has died. First angel told the second one, 'the trader was so rich he had everything even then you mend his wall. But let this poor farmer's goat die, why did you do this?'

The first angel replied, 'things are never the same as they appear.' I had seen you mending the hole of his basement wall,' said the second angel. What is the story behind this?' The first angel said, 'the trader was a very greedy man that is why I tried to mend his basement's wall which had a hole in it. If he would have seen that treasure he would have grown greedier. And if the matter is about this farmer, then know that last night Death came to take his wife but I was sleeping on his wife's bed. So when Death came he was amazed to see me, and told he cannot return empty handed. To that I asked him to take his goat in the place of his wife.' To hear all this, the second angel knew everything now; things are not always like the way they appear.

Moral

Whatever life presents in front of the eyes, it is not true all the time because sometimes it can be distanced from reality.

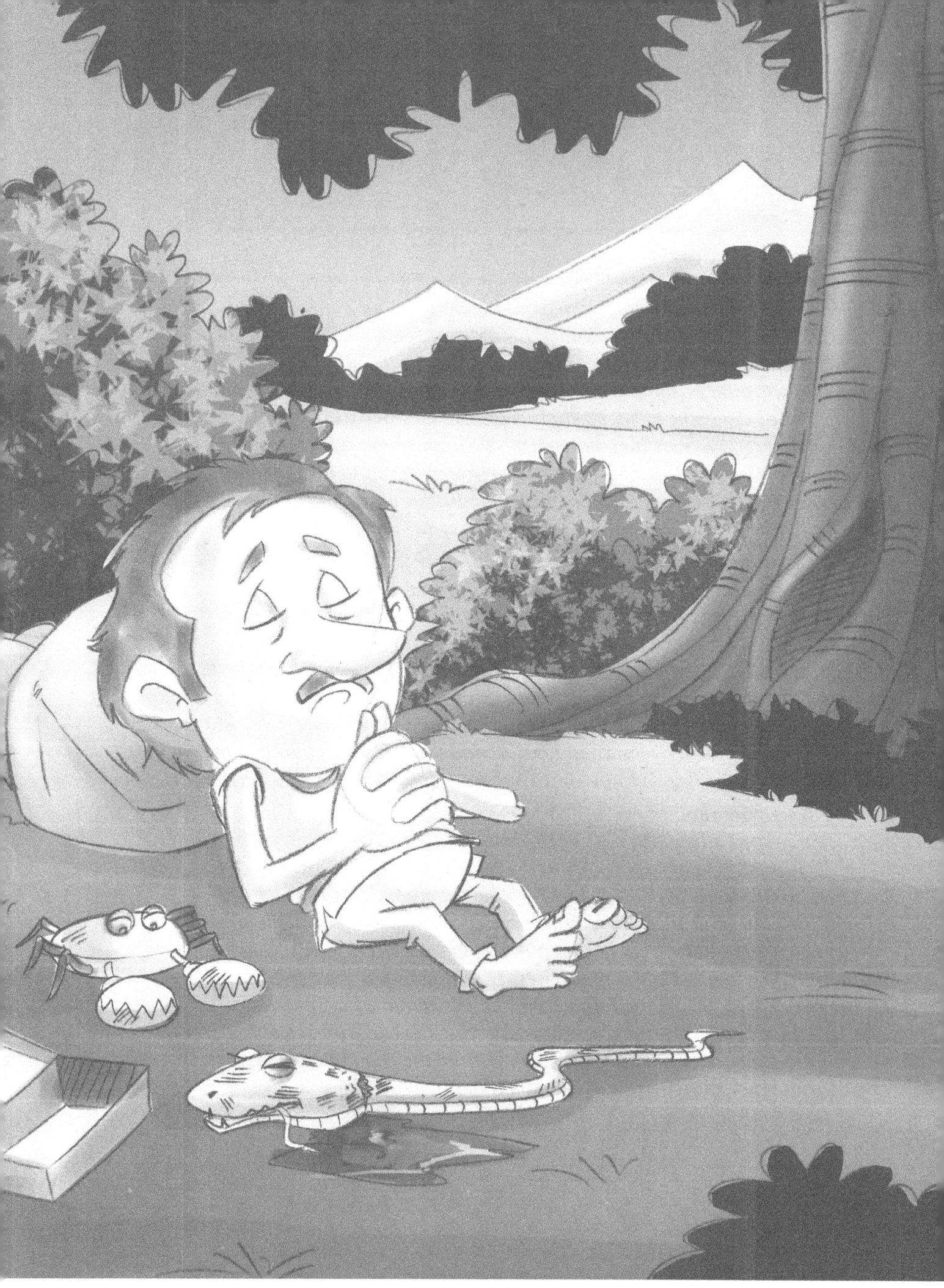

two is better than one

In a village a man lived whose name was Bhola. Once his mother asked him to go someplace for work. She also asked him to take someone with him because he would be crossing the forest. Bola said, 'I will take someone along on the way.' But he did not find anyone who would agree to come with him. Therefore he decided to travel alone. But his mother's instruction was echoing in his head all the time. While walking he picked a crab from the nearby flowing river and kept it safely in a box of camphor and placed it in his bag. He though in his heart, he has followed his mother's instruction and any time two is better in number than one. To be realistic how can a crab help me?

He walked several miles. Now he became tiered of walking. Bhola went under a tree to take a nap. Under the cool shadow of the tree it did not take long for him to fall asleep. Inside the hollow of the tree trunk there lived a fierce snake. To see a person sleep unaware it came out from the hollow to bite. When the snake came closer to Bhola he smelled something nice which was camphor. He was distracted from Bhola now and he was hitting the box of camphor lying in the bag with his fang. When it hit the box with a lot of force then it got broken somehow, and the crab got out and a small piece of this broken box got stuck in the snake's fang. As soon as crab saw this he held the snake with its claws and grabbed its neck. And that snake died. When Bhola woke he saw his box was open and broken and nearby a snake was lying dead with a piece of his box got stuck in his fang. He also saw the crab was roaming at a distance. It did not take him long to understand what his mother meant when she said, when travelling two is always better than one.

It is often said home is not a house or a single town or a map. It is wherever the people who lone you are, whenever you are together.

Moral

One must not travel alone. To be in a company of someone the journey becomes easy and free of hurdles.

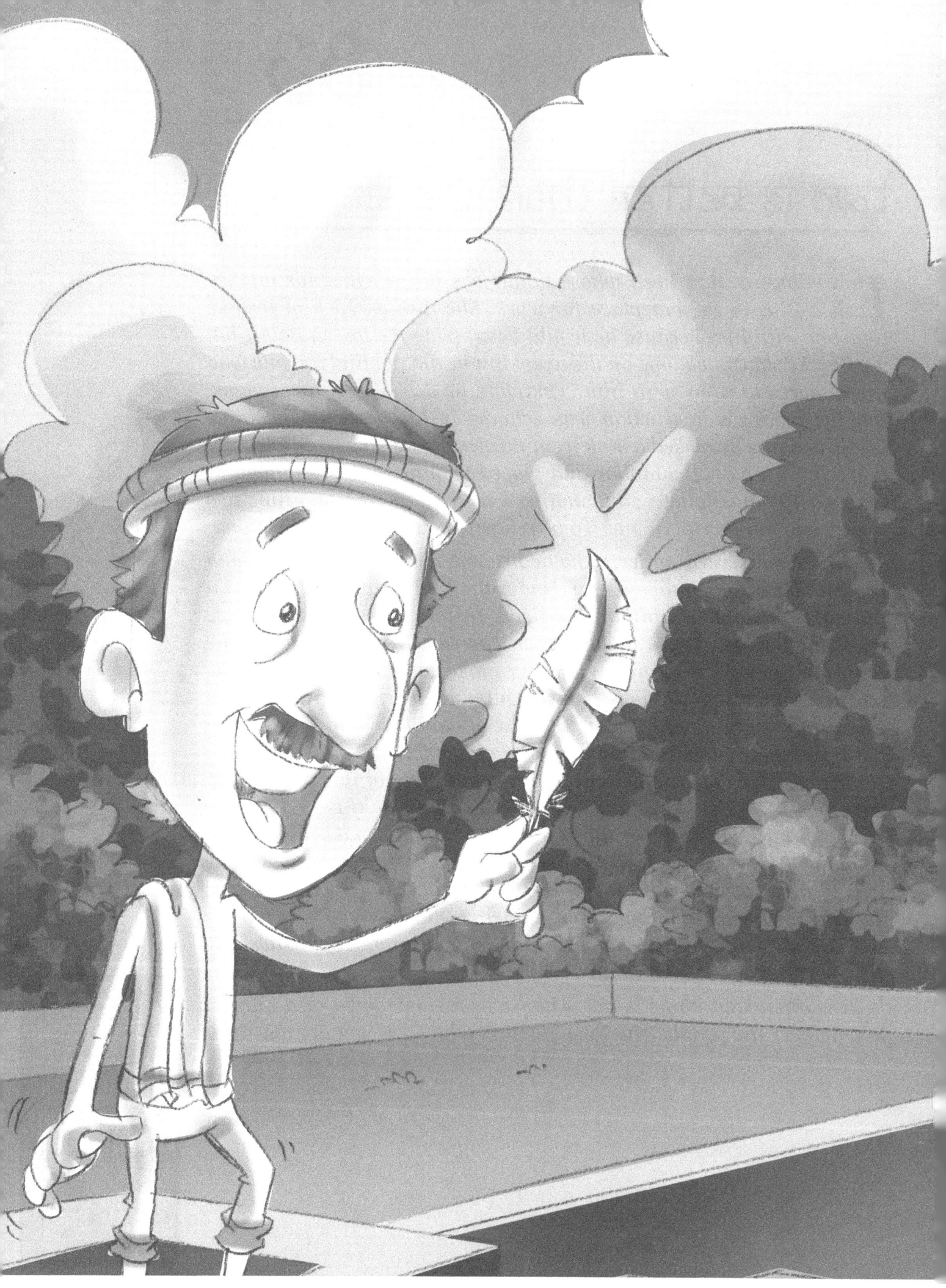

34

bounties of greed

There was a village called Chandanpur where a person named Girdhari used to live. Girdhari was a very virtuous man. His wife Bhagwati would always complain about their poverty but he would never utter a single word which God would disapprove of. One day she started cursing Girdhari that he revres God a lot but does he ever listen to him? Bhagwati had to say just this much, all of a sudden a white swan came flying in and perched in their front yard.

Girdhari tried to caress this white swan and as soon as he did caress it, one of its feathers fell on the ground. Seeing the broken feather which fell from swan's body Girdhari could not believe his eyes. That white swan's broken white feather turned into a gold feather right in front of him. In his heart Girdhari thanked God for his bounty and Bhagwati lifted that feather safely from there. Now this swan started coming every day, Girdhari would caress it lovingly the swan would shed one feather every day which would turn into gold. And Girdhari would give that feather to his wife every day.

One day Bhagwati's heart was filled with greed. Next day as soon as the white swan came she grabbed hold of that bird. Before Girdhari could speak anything she plucked all feathers one by one from that swan's body. Bhagwati saw that swan was hurt and it was covered in blood but not even a single feather turned into gold this time. Within few moments the dying swan said to her, 'this is the reward of greedy people. To attain more, one losses even half of the share or boon.' Bhagwati tried to resuscitate the swan but in vain. She sought the help of Girdhari also but even he couldn't revive the swan. The swan died. Other than remorse there was no way left for Bhagwati in the end.

Moral

Greed brings no reward or bounty with itself.

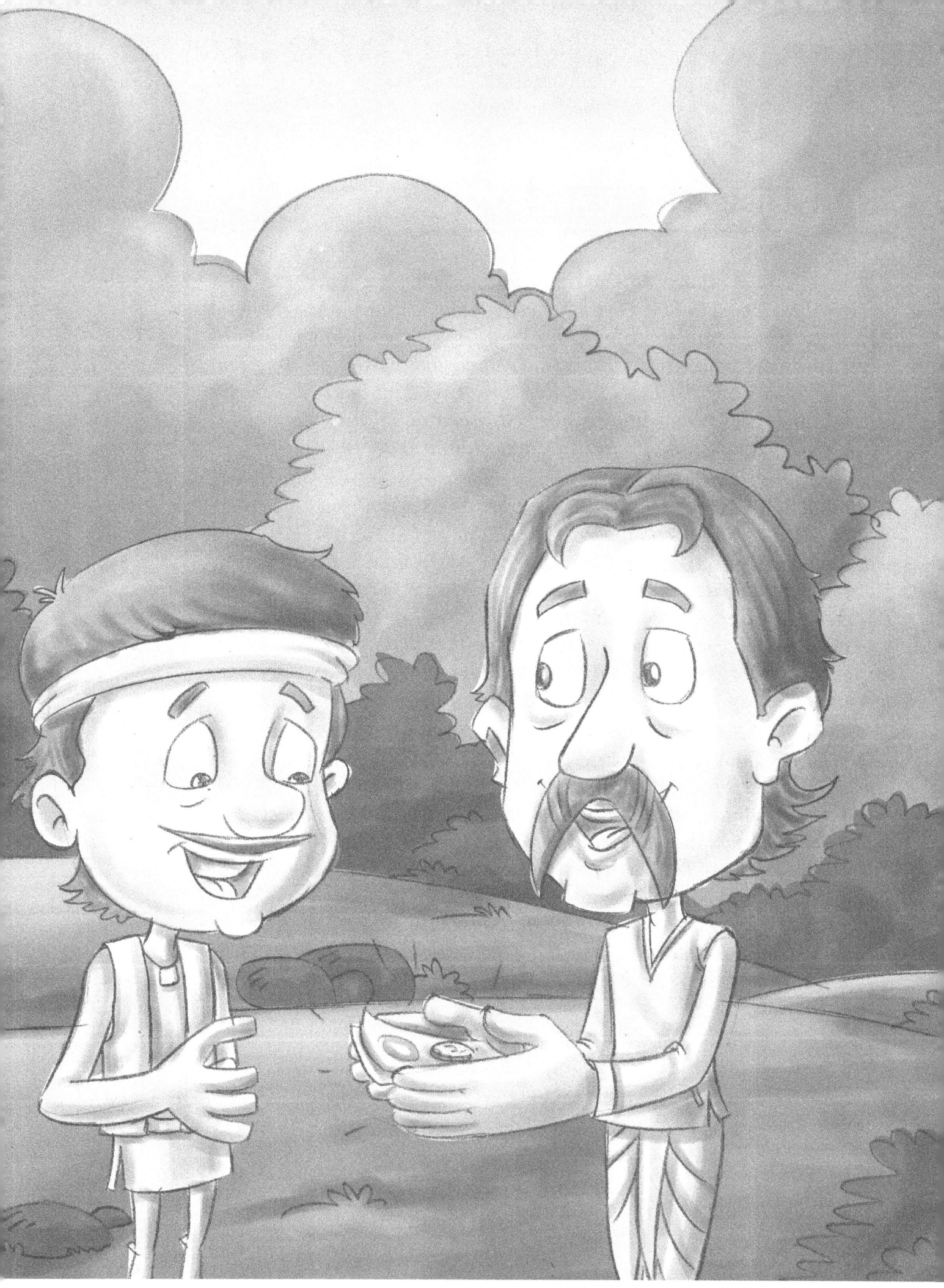

praise to dayaram

In a village lived four good friends. Dayaram was the poorest of them all. One day all four friends decided to go for a bath in the holy river Ganga. To go for a pilgrimage Dayaram had no money for such a journey. His friends told him, 'take money from us you can return us when you come back.' All of them agreed to give him five hundred rupees and went back to their respective homes and started preparing for the journey.

While returning home Dayaram saw a man was dragging a dead donkey to a certain place. Dayaram could not see this happening so he said, 'why are you dragging this poor creature so hard even after his death? And why did you not perform its last rites?' The man replied 'my children are hungry at home, if someone would buy this dead donkey then my children sitting with hunger will get some food to eat.' Dayaram took out all the money from his pocket and gave to the needy person and said 'after performing last rites you will save some money use that for your benefit.'

When all three friends reached Dayaram's house to take him along he refused to go to holy Ganges with them. His friends thought that after getting money he has changed his mind. They cursed him and started their journey to go to the holy river. All along they kept cursing Dayaram. When they reached the Ganges they heard every person praising Dayaram's deed. They were quite amazed because Dayaram never reached the holy river. How come this place was praising him so much?

They stopped one man and asked, 'listen brother! Who is this person called Dayaram and why everyone here is praising him so much?' he replied, 'Who is Dayaram even we do not know but he is one kind hearted man. He has done some really great work because of which his praise and admiration has reached this place also. That is why we are praising him here as well. And whosoever is praised here gets the benefit of bathing in holy water while sitting in his home.' His friends realised their wrong action. They realised their friend's worthiness and praised him as well and completed their holy bath in the water. So it must be true-if your heart is pure then one does not need a dip in the holy waters.

Moral

Nothing is more precious than the lives of living beings, and no ritual- as fast or holy bath is as great as the love for the fellow beings.

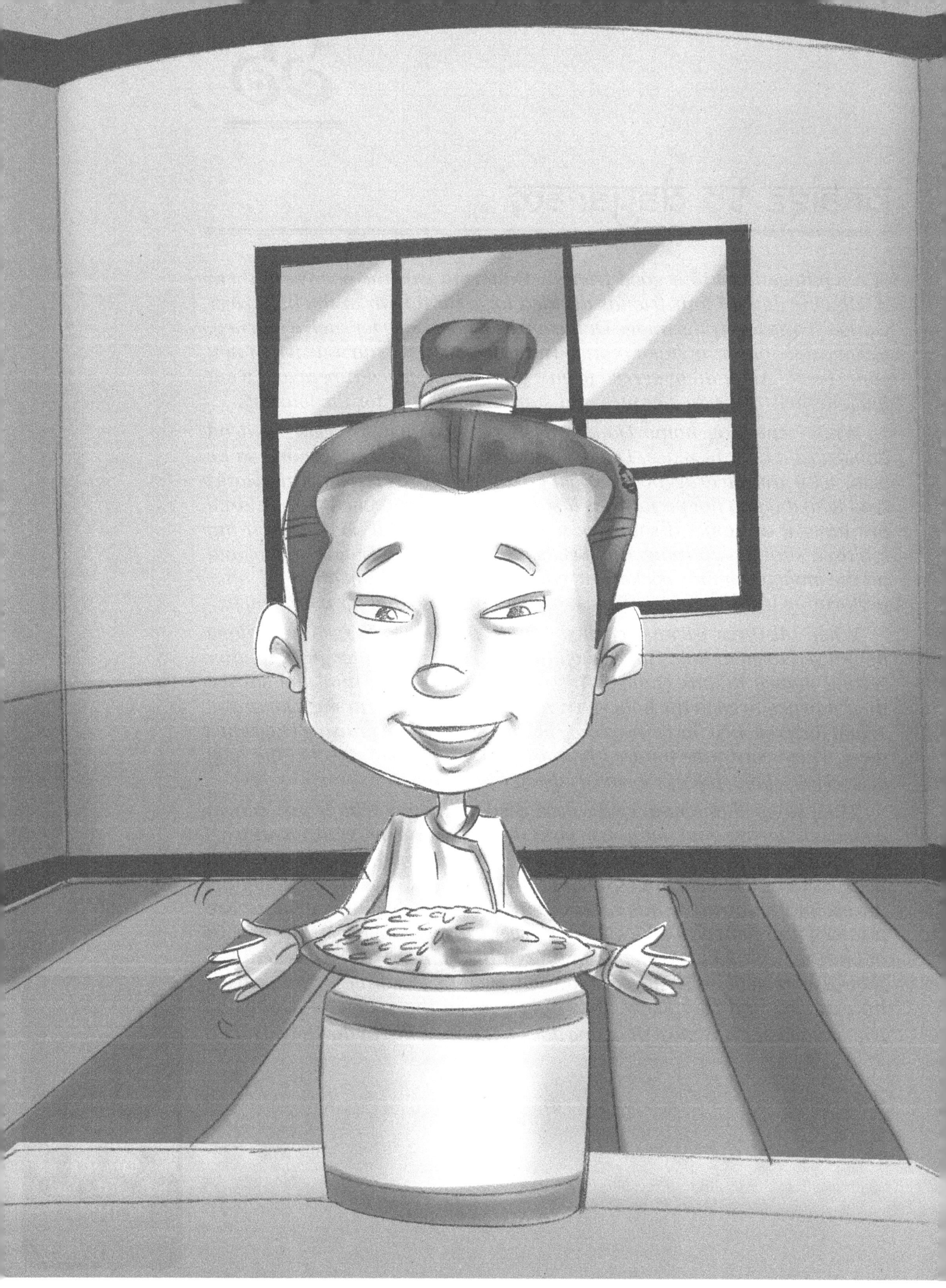

birth of the dragon

*L*ong, long ago a boy named Chi-Yun lived in China. He lived with his mother in a small house. There were greener pastures all around the village. Chi-Yun will go towards his fields every morning. He would chop fresh grass and deliver it to a farmer called Hun-Tsi. He needed fresh grass every day for his cow. In lieu of the grass he would give Chi-Yun a jar of rice every day.

A year went by. There was no rain in the village. All grass turned yellow. Chi-Yun would search for green grass everywhere. A time came when Chi-Yun and his mother had nothing to eat. One day he decided to go beyond those green hills in search of grass. Beyond the hill he saw patchs of grass. Chi-Yun became very happy and started cutting the grass. Next day also he chopped green grass from this place and gave it to Hun-Tsi. Once white chopping grass he saw something gleaming. It was a golden pearl. He picked up the pearl and went home to hide it in the jar of rice. Then a miracle happened. Whenever Chi-Yun would empty his rice jar it will get filled again. Chi-Yun learnt this all was happening because of magic pearl. Now Chi-Yun started sharing the same rice with all his fellow village people. And villagers were very grateful to him. But farmer Hun-Tsi was not happy with all this. He wanted to acquire this golden pearl.

He told Chi-Yun to take all his money, house, fields and wealth but in return give that magical pearl. Chi-Yun said, 'No I cannot give you this magic pearl of mine. It is for the betterment of all villagers.'

One night Hun-Tsi got inside Chi-Yun's house to steal his golden pearl. But somehow Chi-Yun woke up. Hun-Tsi leapt towards his jar. and swallowed the magic pearl after fetching it out of jar. That magic pearl started burning inside his belly. He started feeling thirsty. He drank and finished all the water inside his house. Then he drank water from, pond and river but was still thirsty. He started suffering in pain. After this flames started to come out of his mouth. Hun-Tsi realised his mistake. He left the village, to go beyond those hills never to return back. People say this is how the dragon was born.

Moral
To steal someone's property and make it your own is a major crime, and its punishment can be very horrible.

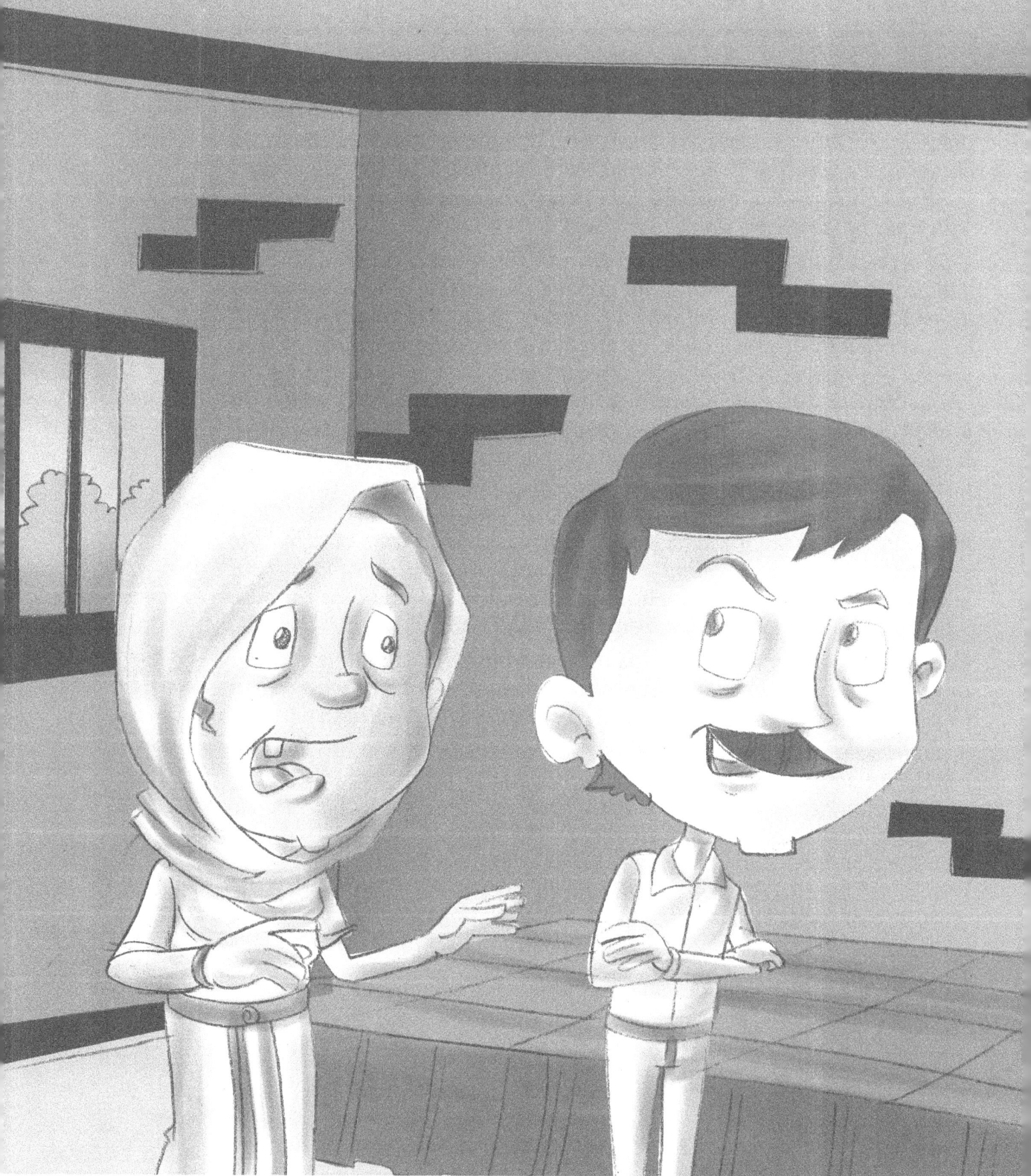

pride

*I*n a city lived a poor woman whose name was Sushila. She also had a son. She educated and raised her son quite well and he grew to be an able person. He became a big employee somewhere. When he attained a higher rank he became very proud of himself. He would not regard anyone greater than him. Whosoever will come to him he would try to look down at him. When Sushila learnt about this habit in her son she felt very sad. One day she tried to tell her son in a loving fashion, 'son! a person who is biggest in this world is the one who considers himself the smallest of the creature present.'

But her son did not regard what she has told him. He was absorbed in his higher position so much. Time changes so fast before one can even know. One day, the son was going someplace and met with an accident and injured his legs badly. Best of the doctors tried to treat his legs but nothing helped and in the end they had to cut his limbs. After few days he was thrown out of his position. Now the son was very worried. His entire pride was shattered into bits. He experienced that life is unpredictable. Just like this it is the same with position and fame or money and wealth together. A person who is proud of his position always falls. Human beings should have self-respect not the self-pride.

Moral

Too much of pride is a way to downfall. That is why never invest oneself in fake glory or pride.

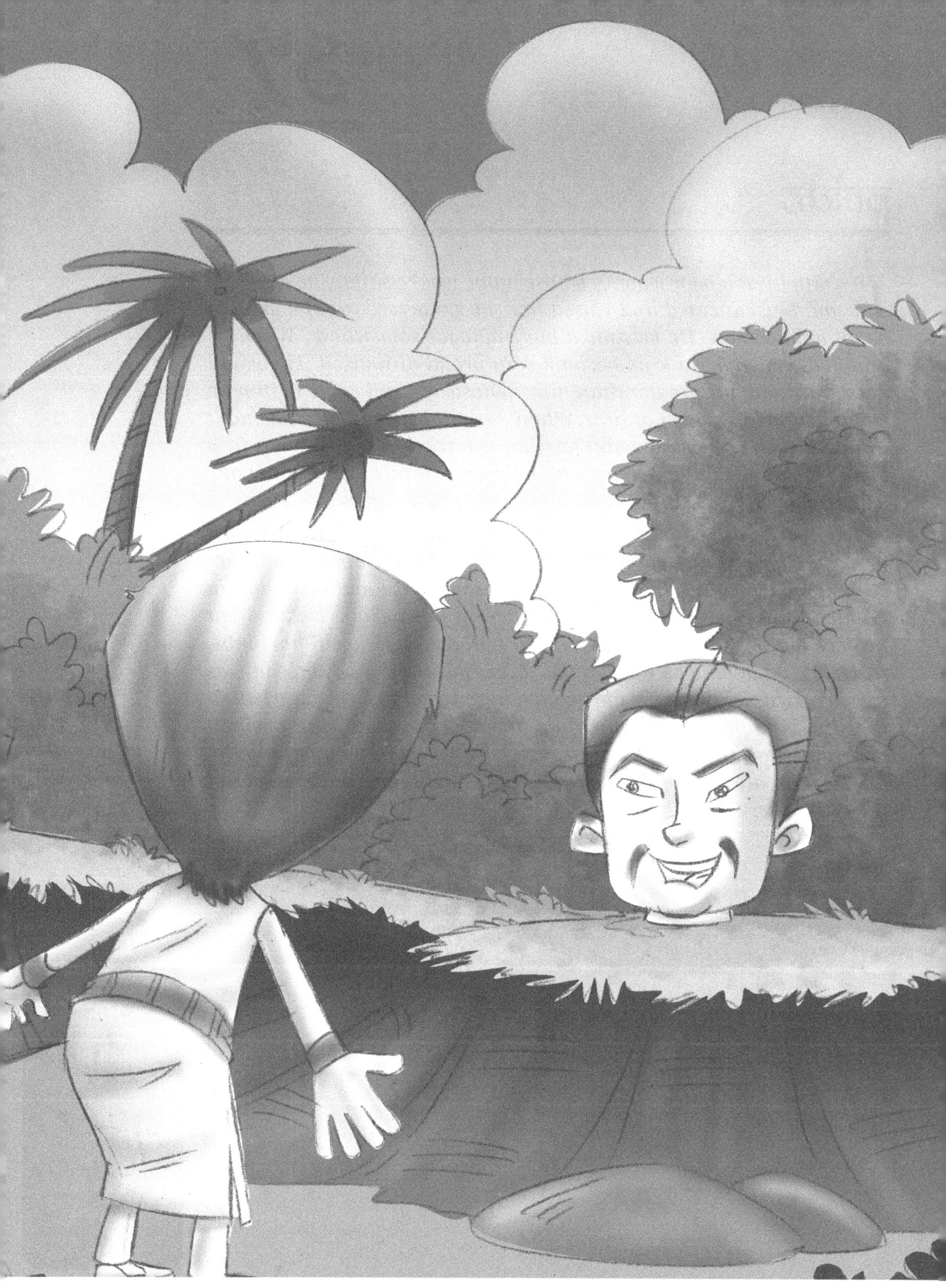

the secret of the coconut tree

*I*n Myanmar a coconut tree is called 'Gaan-bin'. Its meaning is the tree of mischief makers. There is a wonderful story behind it. Many years ago a cruise carrying three people reached the coast of Burma. Burma was previously known as Myanmar. All three people were asked to see the king. It was believed these in three men had committed some crime their own country and had fled here. One of the persons was a thief. The other one was a magician and the third a conspiracy maker.

After listening to three men the king asked his minister to give the thief and the magician one thousand silver coins and permitted them to settle down in Burma. But the king decided to hang the man who was the conspiracy maker. According to the king the thief would steal things from the people, because he was a poor man. And the magician was also poor that is why he would cast spells on people. King spoke about the conspiracy maker, 'that such a person who gets into the act of conspiring never stops, he keeps on churning conspiracies against others.'

The conspiracy maker was taken to the coast and was hanged. Next day one of the king's administrator went where the conspiracy maker was hanged. The head portion of the man who was hanged was lying there. He screamed, 'tell your king to come and bow his head in front of me or else I will break his skull.' Afraid the administrator ran to see the king and said, 'Your Highness, The head of the person who was hanged is lying on the ground and speaking. If you do not believe me send one of your men to testify the truth.' The king sent another administrator with the first one.

When both the men reached the spot, the head did not speak at all. The administrator reported what he saw. In anger king punished the first administrator to be hanged. When the man was to be hanged, the head of conspiracy maker started laughing, 'Ha...ha...ha, I still can churn any conspiracy even after my death.' King felt sad now. Worried that the conspiracy maker's head can create more trouble in his kingdom the king ordered to bury the head in a very deep pit. A tree sprung up the very next day with several fruits on it. The fruits looked like the conspiracy maker's head. It was a coconut tree that people in Burma call it 'the tree of conspiracy maker'.

Moral

The crime of any conspiracy maker is unpardonable.

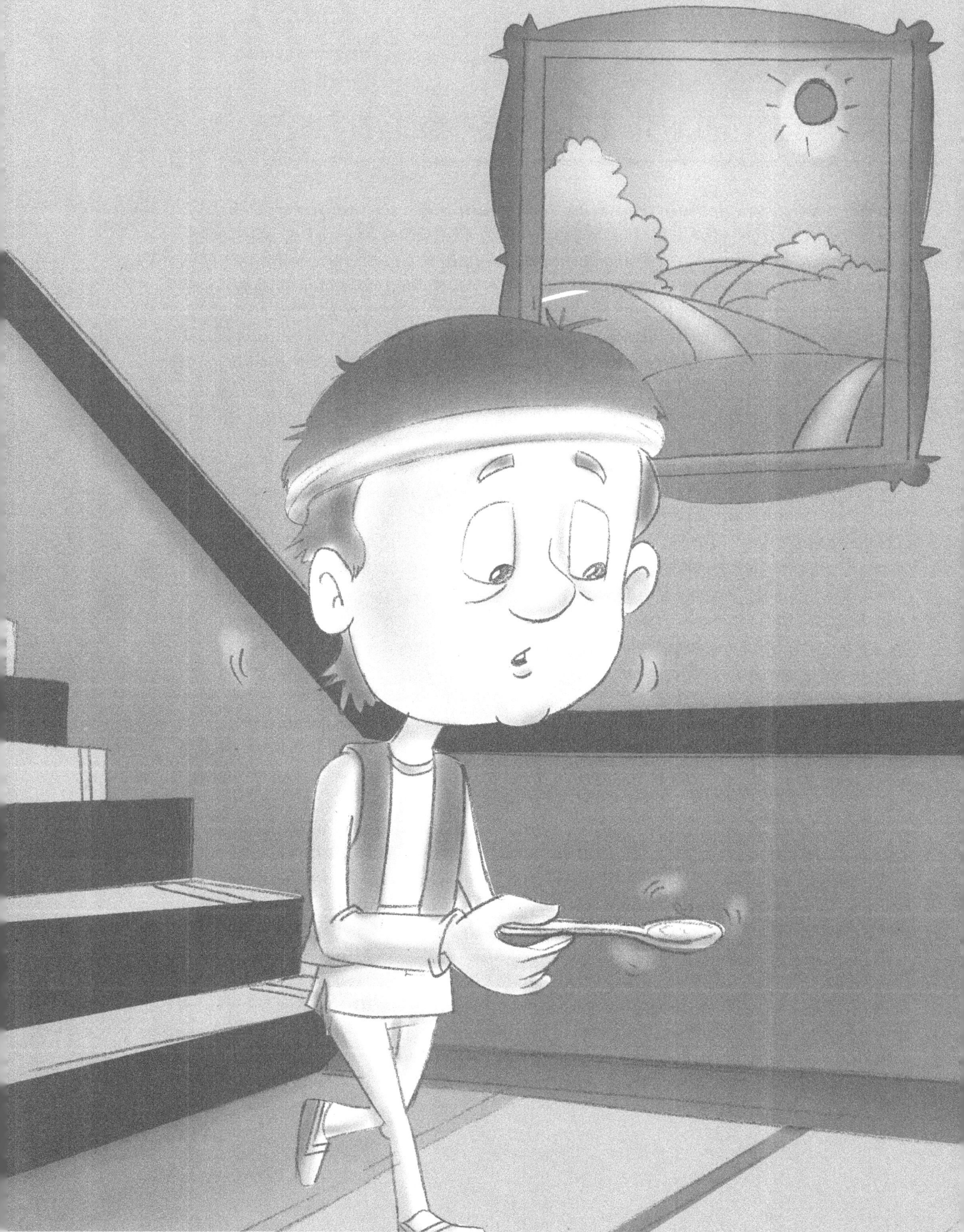

the secret of being happy

One day shopkeeper Shambhu's son Murli asked his father. 'Father what is the secret of being happy forever?' Shambhu replied 'Son on a mountain far from here there is a palace. A man lives there. Only he can answer this question.' After walking for so long he saw the mountain and the palace on it. When he entered this palace he saw many people were surrounding an attractive but stern looking man and seeking solutions to their queries. They were calling him 'Your Highness.' To meet him Murli had to wait for two hours. 'His Royal Highness listened to the reason of Murli's coming there and said, 'I do not have time to answer your question right now. Come after two hours. Meanwhile you can see my palace and roam around.' When Murli was leaving this place His Highness gave him a spoon and added two drops of oil in it and said 'be careful so that while walking you do not drop anything from it.'

Murli climbed many stairs up and down but he did not keep his eyes away from that spoon for a single moment. After two hours he returned back to His Highness. He asked Murli, 'did you see a beautiful painting hanging in my room? Did you also see my vast garden? And have you seen all the books lying in my library?' But Murli was quite ashamed he told His Highness that he could not concentrate on anything other than this spoon and two drops of oil in it that is why he could not see anything else. To that His Highness replied, 'then go and see everything carefully in my palace.' Now Murli went and saw everything kept in this palace carefully and enjoyed each and every detail thoroughly. After returning he explained the Royal Highness in detail. After listening to Murli he asked him 'tell me where is that drop of oil which I gave you?' When Murli looked at the spoon there was no drop of oil in it. The Royal Highness spoke 'this is the secret of being happy, which remains in seeing and enjoying everything of this world but never to forget that drop of oil which one contains always.'

Moral

The secret of being happy is to enjoy life to the fullest, but one must always concentrate on God.

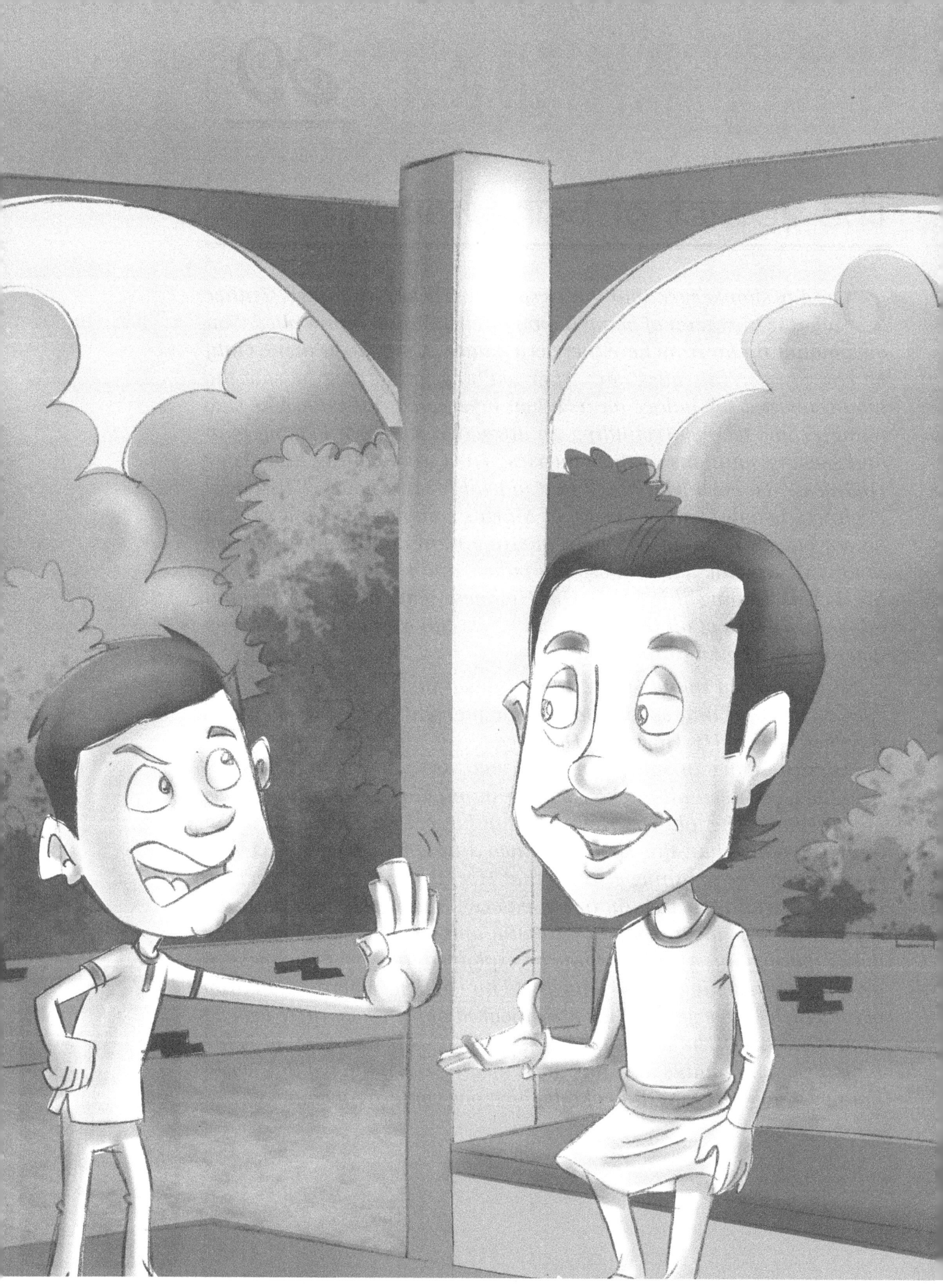

40

Repentance

It was one such morning. When Budhiprakash was sitting outside his house with his parents and was having his morning tea. All of a sudden a crow came flying towards his veranda. To see that crow father asked his son 'what is that?' Budhiprakash said softly 'it is a crow father.' After a lot of time he asked again 'what is this creature?' Budhprakash said 'it is a crow.' But some time later father asked the same question again 'what is this?' Budhiprakash replied in a very loud voice 'it is a crow how many time do I have to tell you the same thing.'

But his father had a disease where he tends to forget a lot. And forth time he directed his finger towards crow and said the same thing, 'Son what is this?' But now Buhiprakash could not take his question further, he got up very frustrated, and said 'Father this is the limit how many times you will ask the same question? I am tired of repeating this answer but you are not tired of asking it.' Budhiprakash's mother was sitting next to him and she was listening to all this. She was sitting right next to him, and said-'when you were really small, then you used to ask the same question from your father repeatedly just like this. This is how you used to ask about a bird once. That too not even once or twice but twenty or thirty times in a row. But I do not remember that your father replied in anger not even once. All the time he told you lovingly that son it is a bird. And now that he has a habit of forgetting you are getting angry after replying to him after four attempts.' After listening to his mother's remarks he felt ashamed and it can be seen in his eyes. He asked for apology from his father immediately.

These days youngsters are getting impatient and intolerant in their attitude. They are also becoming less respectful to elders. This is creating problems not only in the society but within family itself. So we have to be careful about how we behave with our elders otherwise our children will also treat us in the same manner when we become old.

Moral

One must not get agitated with the elders' remarks or queries.

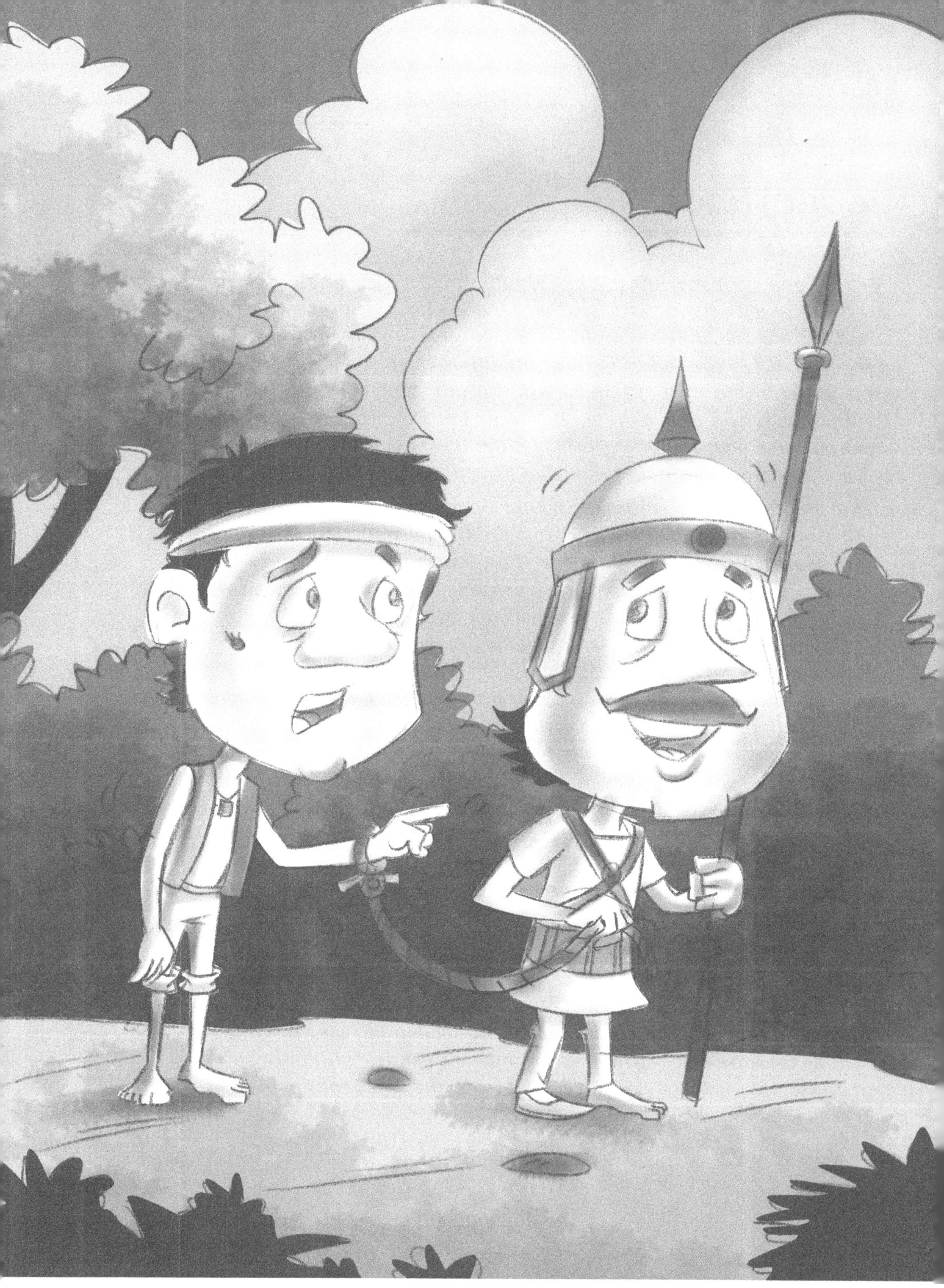

god will give more

One of the king's soldiers was chasing a thief. He was riding his horse with fast speed. He realised his shoe has fallen when he was in full galore of riding his horse. Without being bothered about his fallen shoe he kept going straight ahead in his speed. Someone screamed from behind, 'Oh brother! Your shoe has fallen. At least pick it up.' This horse rider while speeding on his horse yelled back at the person, 'God will give more.' While galloping the horse leapt from all bushes and hurdles but the rider's turban got stuck on the branch of a tree when his horse was unable to leap from a branch of tree hanging mid-way.

Then again someone saw this and screamed to inform him, 'Listen brother! You turban is stuck.' The soldier replied again, 'God will give more.' This was heard even by the thief who was running ahead of him. Within no time the soldier grabbed hold of that thief. When soldier was returning back after catching this thief he witnessed a different scene on his way. One man was walking with his shoes worn not in his feet but he was holding them in his hands. Then this thief asked soldier, 'why is this man not walking with his shoes in his feet but held them in his hands? He thinks that his shoes will be torn and god will not give him another pair of shoes. Then why you keep on saying "God will give more"?' soldier laughed and said both the things are very different. 'He is walking on the track of selfhood and when I lost my things I was performing my duty. I walk on the track of my duty with the assurance of god but this fellow is walking on the path governed by his self-absorbed nature.' Now this thief understood when walking the track of duty all attachments get lost in performing duty selflessly, and all material objects cannot be a hindrance in performing a bigger task.

It is said that self-less duty calls for you to sacrifice your own worldly needs and do whatever it takes to protect the interest of the world.

Moral

People who follow their duty they do not attach themselves to all worldly objects and materials.

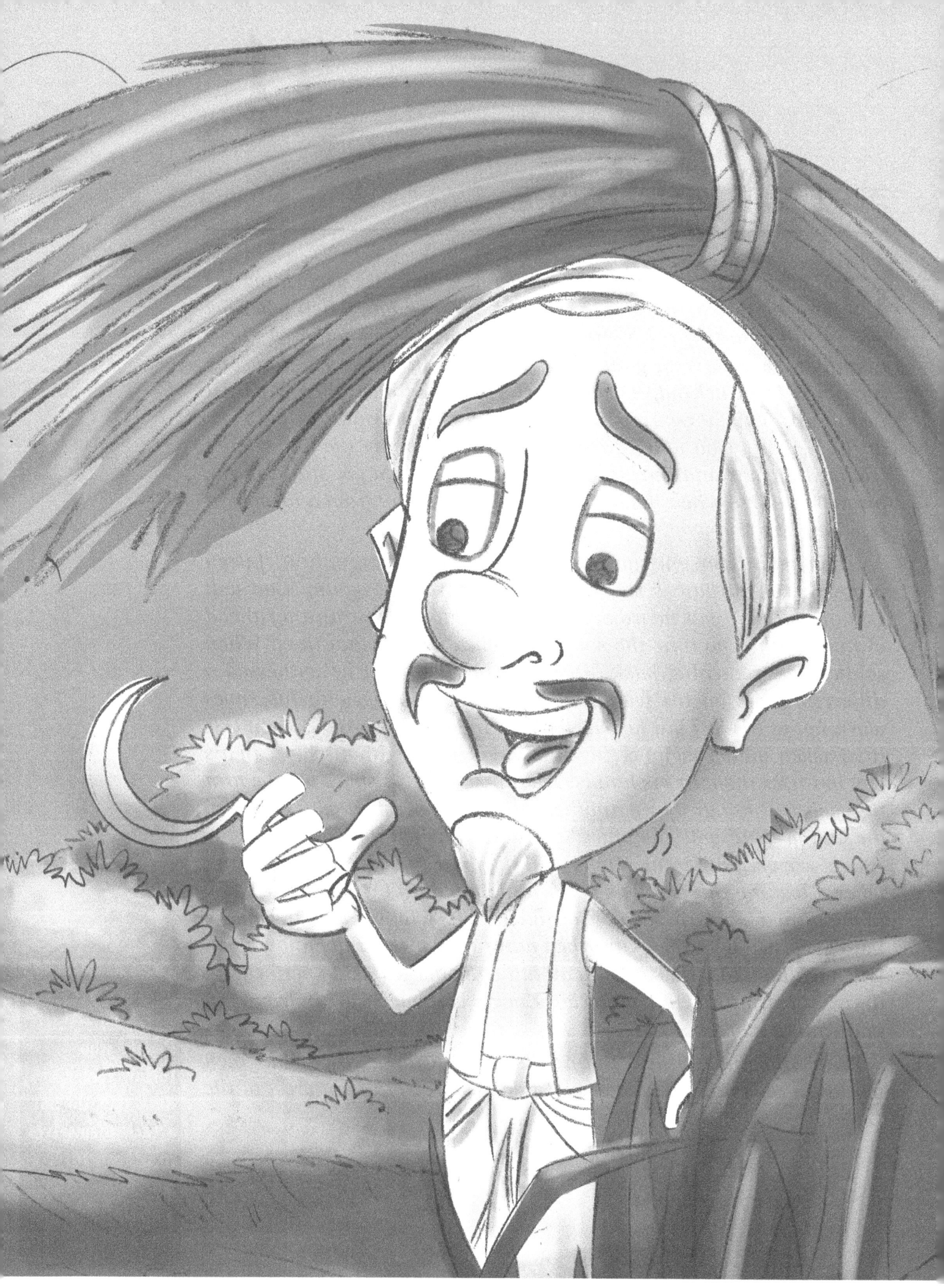

sheikchilli's cure

Sheikchilli used to go to the forest every day to cut fresh grass. One day after cutting the grass he was returning home, he realised his grass reaper was left behind in the forest. He went back to the forest to get back his grass reaper. Due to scorching sun the reaper had become quite hot to touch. As soon as Shekchilli touched it his hand could feel its heat. He thought the grass reaper has got a fever. He took it to a doctor and said 'Oh doctor! I think my grass reaper has got a fever kindly prescribe some medicine for it.' Doctor thought that Sheikchilli was playing a prank on him. He touched the reaper and said, 'Yes it has got fever. Tie it with a rope and hang it inside a well, all its fever will get down'. Sheikchilli did the same as he was told by the doctor. The reaper was cold to touch after getting drowned in water and Sheikchilli thought doctor's advice finally worked.

One day an old woman living in Sheikchilli's neighbourhood got fever. When her family members were taking her to see the doctor he said 'why are you all taking her to the doctor what treatment he will tell I can prescribe it here only. Just make him deep in some small well on pound. Her fever will be gone. Doctor himself told me this trick.' People believed Sheikchilli and made the old woman take several dips in a pond. After some time when they touched the old woman's body she was cold and she was dead. Old woman's family members were angry at Sheikchilli and they started to scream at him. Then he said, 'I told you all her fever would go away so it has gone. Now the old woman is cold then why are you all screaming at me. Whatever you want to say, complain it to doctor. It is his treatment anyways.' All the people approached the doctor and they were extremely angry. After listening to them doctor started to beat his head. And he said 'I have prescribed this treatment for Sheikchilli's hot grass reaper, so that it gets cold. But that old lady was a human being not a reaper. You should have got her here for treatment.' For this act of his Sheikchilli had to bear their anger and spite both at the same time. And he has sworn not to tell anyone any kind of treatment to an ailing person.

> **Moral**
>
> Overconfidence is always useless a knowledge which can bring a lot of disrespect as well.

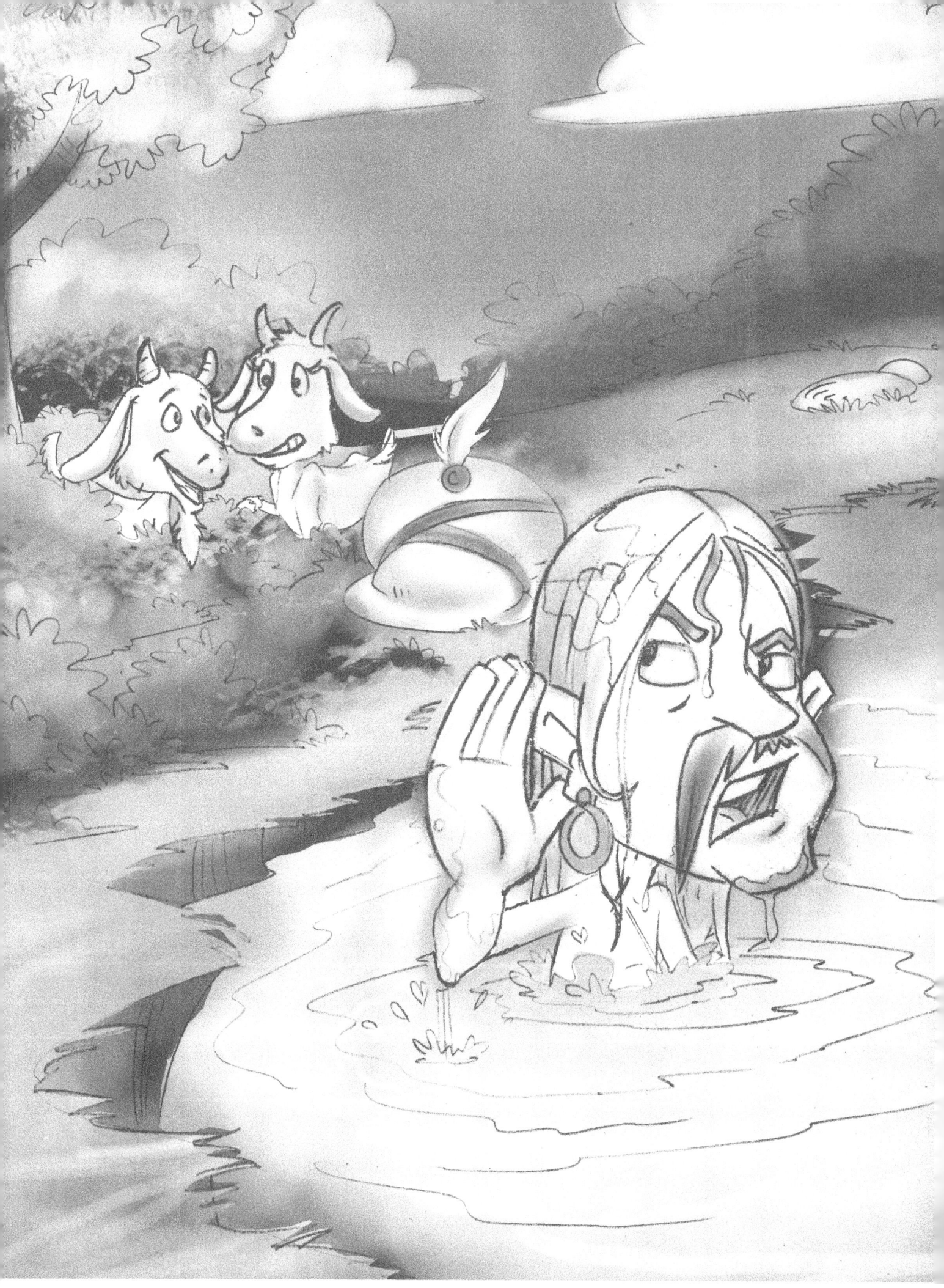

king was saved from his misfortune

Vijaypur's king Kanker Bhagvan was a great follower of Lord Shiva. He prayed Lord Shiva for twenty years. God became happy with him and asked him to demand one blessing as he desired, and the king asked 'I want an ability to understand the languges of all living beings.' To that Lord Shiva said 'that is alright but I also have a condition for you. If you will tell about this boon to any one you will become a stone that very moment.' Lord Shiva gave him this boon and vanished from there.

One day king was having his food. His queen Sumitra was sitting next to him and she was fanning him. Suddenly an ant and a fly arrived there. They both were discussing something about food. The ant said, 'behold yourself fly, you always sit at dirty places. So do not dirty on this food and dirty it.' To that fly said 'why do you think you are so neat and clean? You go anywhere smelling food and waste a lot after eating it. And if you will climb on king's platter then nothing will be worse than me.' To have heard both of them fight king could not help but laughed out loud. The queen saw him laughing insolently. She felt he was humiliating her. She asked him, 'is there something wrong with the food I prepared for you because of which you are laughing?'

King thought if he tells her the truth he will be cast into stone. So let me tell her the truth on the banks of Ganga River so that I will remain there and my life will be complete. He left with the queen for bathing in Ganga. After sometime he came across the river and started to inspect it. He saw the flow of this river. Nearby a male and female goat were talking. Female goat was telling this to the male, 'I feel like having fresh green grass. Can you bring such a grass from the other side of the river?' To this male goat replied 'I am not king Kanker who will give up his life due to his wife's demand. I will slip in the river and I will lose my life. If I were be the king I would have lashed the queen with five hunters and all her demands would have vanished.'

King found goat's remark valid. When he returned to his palace he started to hit her with hunter. Queen started to scream. She said 'it is enough king! From now onwards I will not ask for anything.' King got into trouble due to his secret desire about knowing the animal language also.

Moral

One must never present any form of knowledge in front of a foolish or stubborn person because it may cause a big loss.

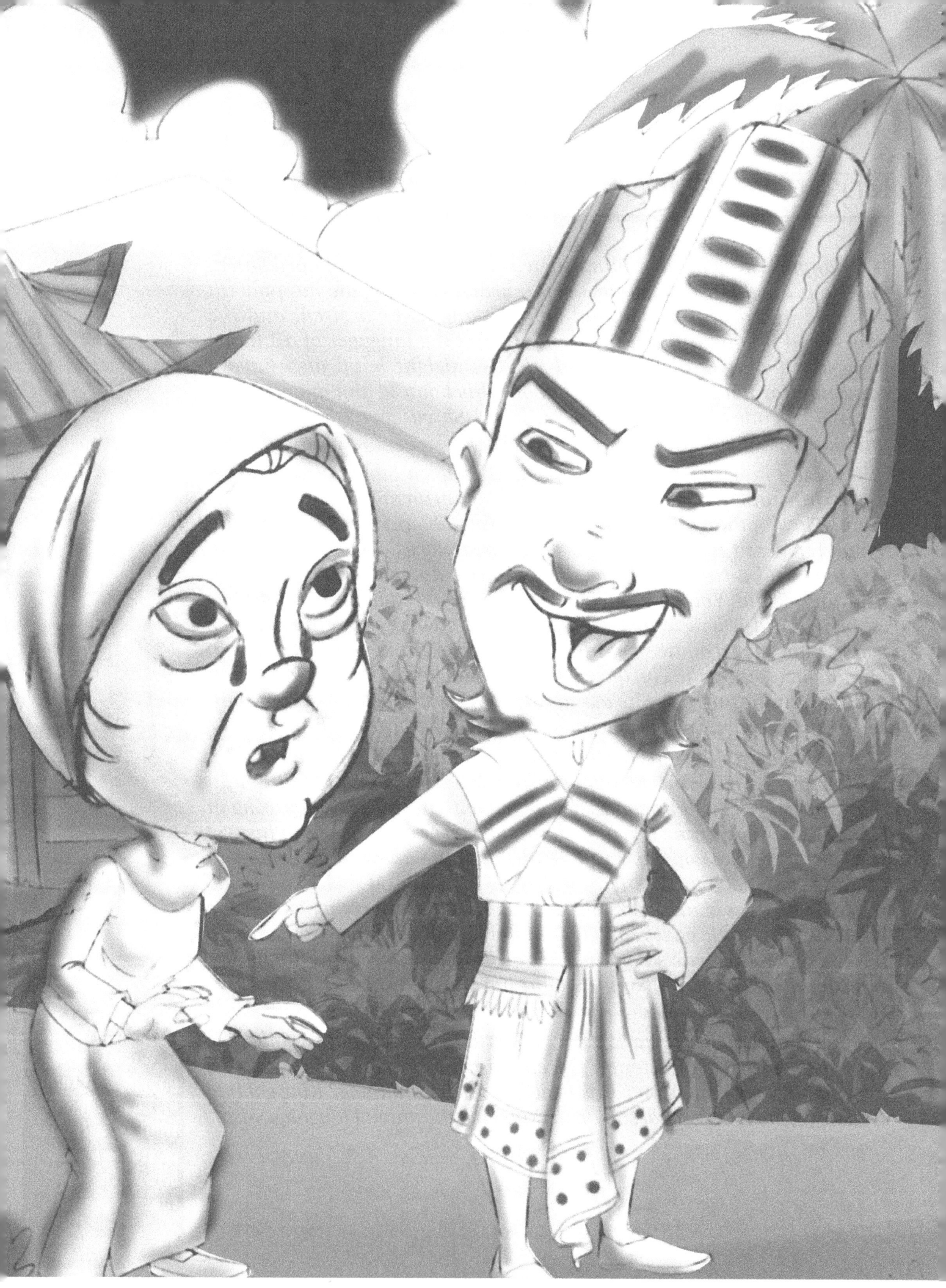

importance of mother

A long, long time ago, in a village in Western Sumatra a woman lived with her son. Malin Kundang. When Malin was very young his father passed away. Since then both mother and son survived in extreme difficulty. Malin was a hardworking and brave boy. He would catch fish every day from sea and give it to his mother. One day when he was trying to catch fish, he saw, a trader's boat attacked by pirates. Malin reached traders boat the point. With his courage and strength he fought and made all the pirates run away. The trader was very happy with Malin and asked him to accompany him on a foreign trade. Malin agreed. The trader made Malin his partner as well. He even got him married to his daughter. Now Manil earned a huge ship, a lot of trading goods with a lot of hands on deck. All these extravagance of life made him a very proud person. One day his ship settle down at the coast near his village. His village people recognised him and soon the news of his arrival spread across his village that Malin Kundang has become a very rich person. When his mother received this news she ran towards the coast to see her son.

This old woman tried three times to meet her son. He yelled at her and refused to see her. I do not have a mother who is old, ugly and haggard like a servant.' He asked his fellow shipmen to take the ship further. She was heartbroken. She cursed him if her son does not seek her forgiveness he will turn into stone.

In a quite sea a turbulent storm broke. Malin's huge vessel was broken into pieces. But it was too late for Malin to realise his mistake and he could not seek his mother's forgiveness. Huge waves threw him away from his ship. He somehow reached towards a small island and turned into a stone.

Moral

The one who insults his mother bears her curse and God punishes such a person in the worst form.

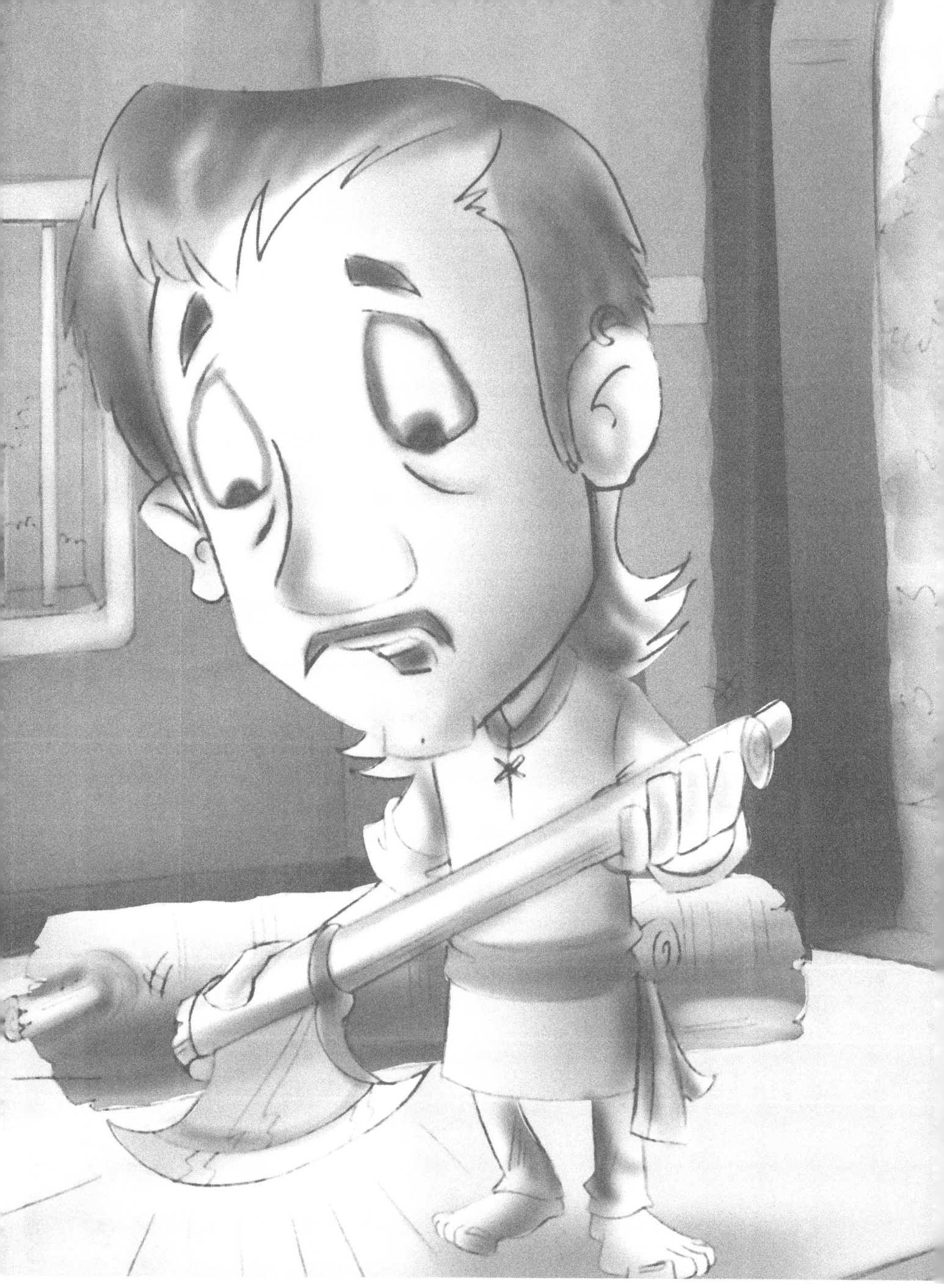

knowledge of misconduct

There was a wood cutter. His name was Shamu. He would chop wood from the forest and sell them in market every day. Whatever money he earned during the day he would sustain his family on that money. One day while he was leaving for the forest to get the wood he looked for his axe all over his house but he could not find it. Another wood cutter used to live right next to his house whose name was Moti. He suspected him for stealing his axe from him because whenever he would look at Moti he could attain through his bare face that the knowledge of misconduct written all over it. For a lot of time not being able to chop woods there was not even a single grain of rice in his home. Neither he had had money to buy a new axe for himself. All day and night he would curse Moti for it.

One day Shamu was moving a huge trunk from his house. Suddenly his eyes got hold of an axe lying next to the trunk. The lost axe was found in his own house. That day when Shamu saw Moti he could not sense the same knowledge of misconduct in in his demeanour or face or in his talk any more. He realised that to know the truth one must keep all windows of possibility open in one's own mind. He asked for forgiveness from God.

From this story we learn that honesty has its own rewards and that honesty is the best policy.

Almost any difficulty will move in the face of honesty and truthfulness when are is honest he would never feel stupid. And when are is honesty, humbleness comes automatically.

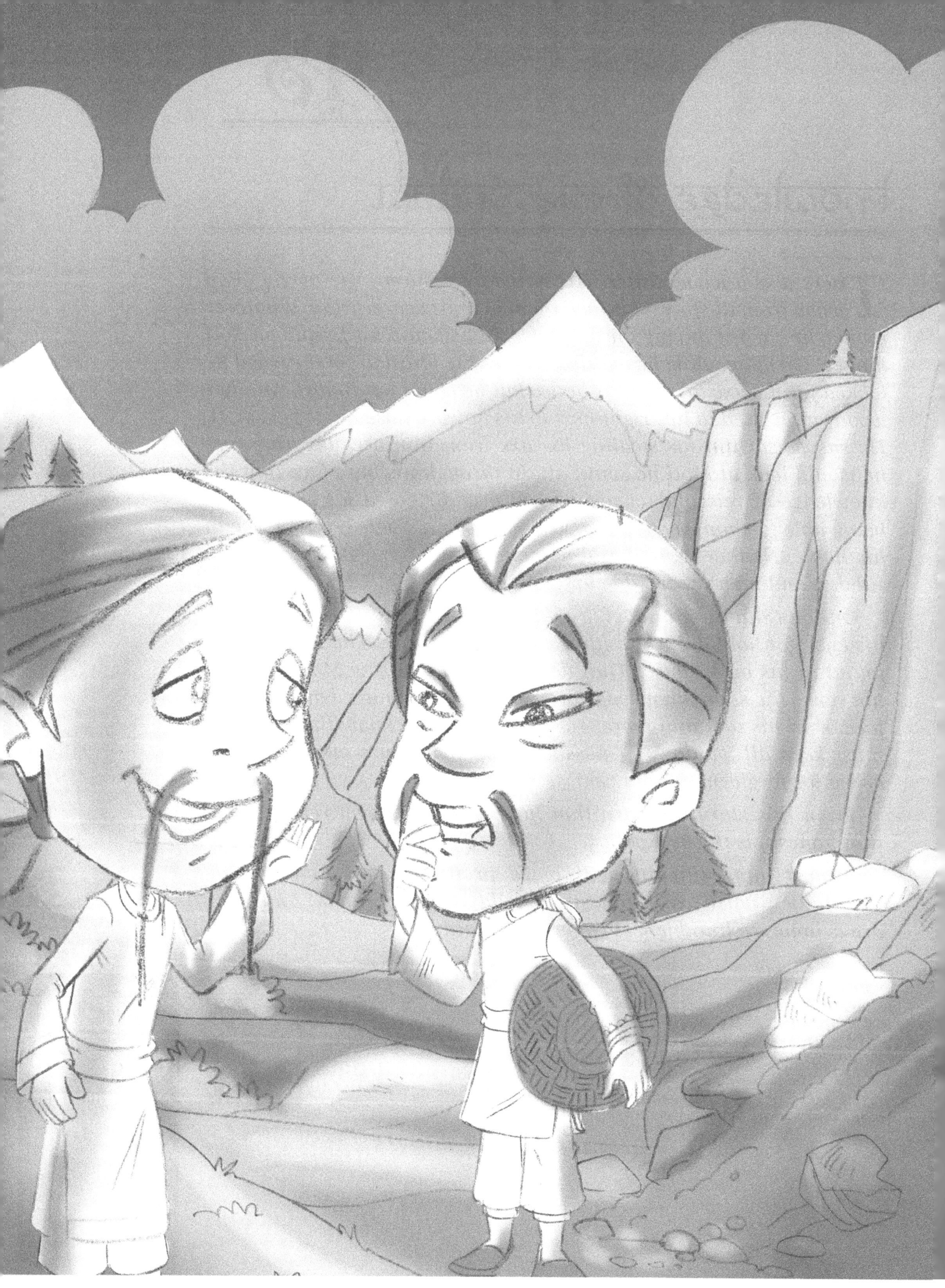

solution of a problem

There was a person named Tai. His house was located on a huge mountain. Any guest who would come to see him had to take a longer route circling the mountain to reach his place. Tai said to his family that he will find a solution for his problem and said, 'we must cut the mountain from its edges every day little by little. One day the entire mountain will be chiselled and we will have a passage through it. Then we or our guests will not have any difficulty in travelling.' His family agreed with Tai's suggestion.

Next day Tai started to cut the mountain with his family's help. Those were the hot summer days. They all would be drenched in sweat but still worked all day and night. Many days were gone and so far they could work on the limited area of the mountain which was cut.

One day Tai's friend Lao came to see him. When he saw Tai's family breaking the mountain he was stunned to see them work on it. He asked, 'what you all are doing here?' To this Tai responded 'we are trying to break this mountain so that people who come up here do not have to walk all around this mountain in order to come here. And if there will be a straight track then people could walk up here easily.' Having heard him speak Lao said 'you all can break such a huge mountain to pave a way for yourself and others it would be better if you can make a house for yourself on the other side of the valley rather than trying to cut through a huge mountain. You and your guests will not have any troubles coming here.'

Tai liked his friend Lao's suggestion and started to work on it immediately. Within few days Tai constructed a new house on the other side of the mountain. His troubles vanished away. It is wisely said if there is big hurdle ahead to solve it one must adopt an easier solution.

We all seem farsighted. We give importance to those things that are far from us, while neglecting the things that are close to us...only to realize their value later when they are out of reach again.

Moral

To solve one problem there are several ways to it. One must adopt a simple and easy way to find a solution

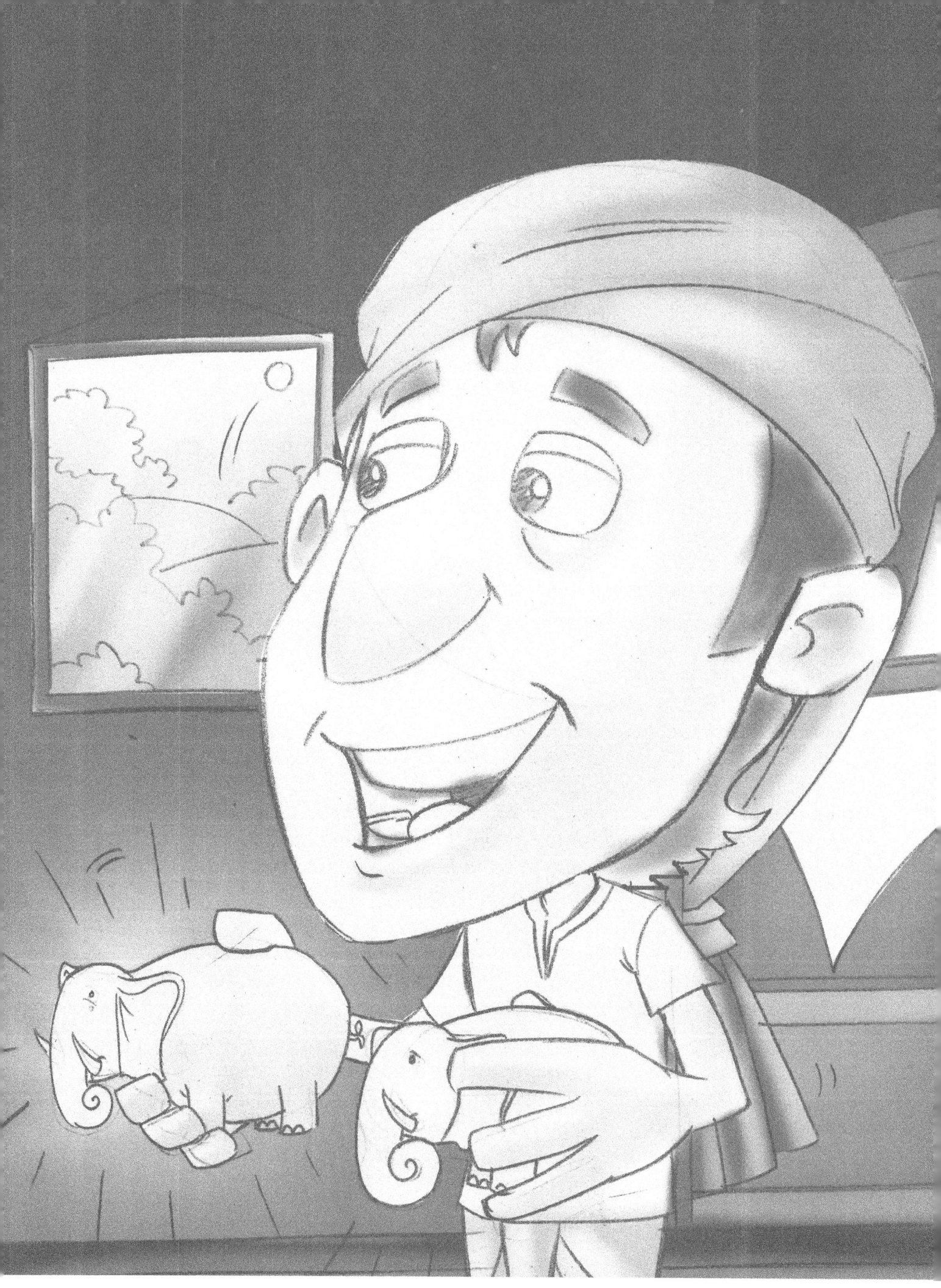

an honest goldsmith

*I*n a village lived a goldsmith. His name was Dhanpat. He had four sons. One day he called all his four sons and asked them 'could you tell me what is an honest goldsmith like?' His elder son said, 'the one who saves four paise out of every rupee.' The second son said 'a true gold smith is that one who makes fifty rupees as his profit and gives the same to his customer.' Third son replied, 'a true gold smith is that one who makes eight paise out of every rupee'. And the forth son replied, 'a true goldsmith is that one who makes a rupee as his profit but keeps his customer happy as ever.'

One trader was listening to their discussion and decided to talk to the youngest son. He asked, 'can you prove your definition of the honest gold smith?' The son replied 'yes I can.' The trader asked him to make a golden elephant for him but only at his house. The goldsmith's son agreed.

From next day onwards he went to trader's house to make that golden elephant. Every day he would return home and make a similar elephant with of brass. When the golden elephant was complete the gold smith's son said 'Sir your golden elephant is ready. But some curd is needed to make it shine.' Right then the trader heard a milkmaid selling curd and decided to buy it. Goldsmith's son said, 'Sir why are you buying curd? Give a little bit more money to this milkmaid I will dip this golden elephant in her pot of curd itself'. And he did.

The trader was quiet happy. He said, I see your definition turned out to be wrong because the elephant is mine and the happiness as well.' Then goldsmith's son said, 'I have not said something false. The milkmaid was my wife and now the real elephant has gone to my house. What you have in your hand is a fake elephant coated with a gold polish. I had dipped the real elephant in the pot of curd but took out a fake one. You became happy to see this one. Then gold smith's son said 'please do not be worried I have done all this to prove my definition right. If I wanted I could have hidden the truth from you. I do not want to be a fraud.' He went to his home and returned trader's real golden elephant to him.

Moral

One must never use one's talent for wrong means.

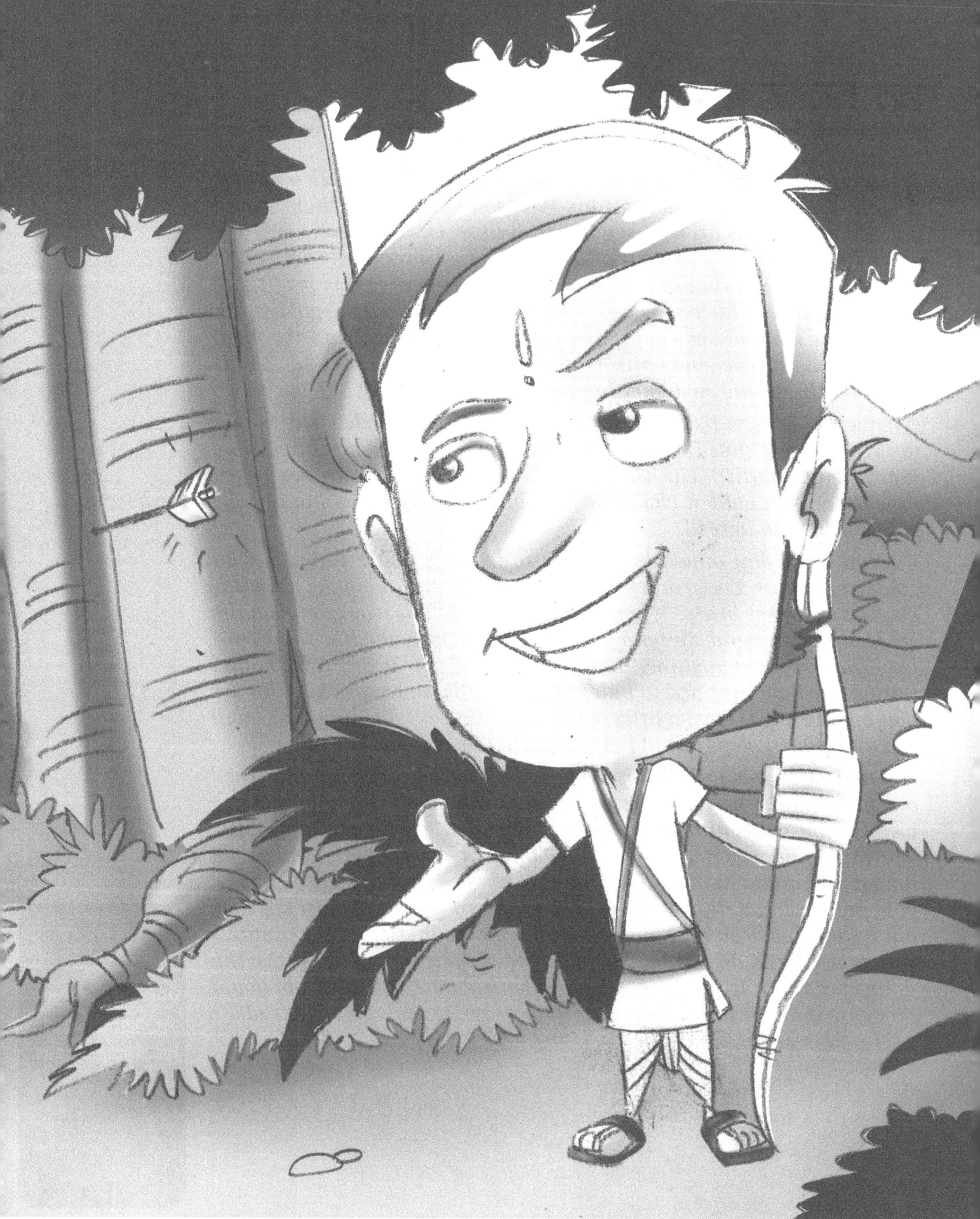

a proud archer

After winning a lot of archery competitions a student fell victim of his own pride and challenged his own teacher in a competition. And his teacher has accepted his challenge.

To show his ability the student was flaunting his archery skill by aiming at a tree. The first arrow hit the point and he shot the second one as well which slit the previous arrow hitting the tree. Then with a lot of pride he said to his teacher 'now show us your skill.'

The teacher asked his student to follow him towards a mountain which was quite large. The student could not understand what was his teacher wanting to do. After climbing the mountain they reached a point from where they could see a deep valley between two mountains. There was a delicate bridge made up of ropes, which appeared quite weak. Due to strong wind this bridge was shaking. The teacher went right in the middle of the bridge and aimed at a tree which was at a longer distance from that point. And his arrow did hit the exact target.

The teacher said to his student, 'now it is your turn. Your arrow should hit closer to my arrow.' After saying it he stood aside.

To see the moving bridge the student was fearful. After a lot of effort he somehow managed to reach right in the middle of it. But he was extremely nervous and he was sweating profusely. Because of his sweaty palms his arrow slipped towards a wrong target and fell in the valley.

As soon as his eyes met his teacher's eye he fell ashamed of his act. Then his teacher said,

'There is no doubt that you are one of the best archers. But you have no balance on your heart's desire, which guides the arrow from any diversion.' The student asked for forgiveness from his teacher and wowed to never ever get influenced by pride.

Wisdom ceases to be wisdom when it becomes too proud to weep, too grave to laugh, and too selfish to seek other than itself.

Moral

To be proud in front of the wisest will cause embarrassment to only.

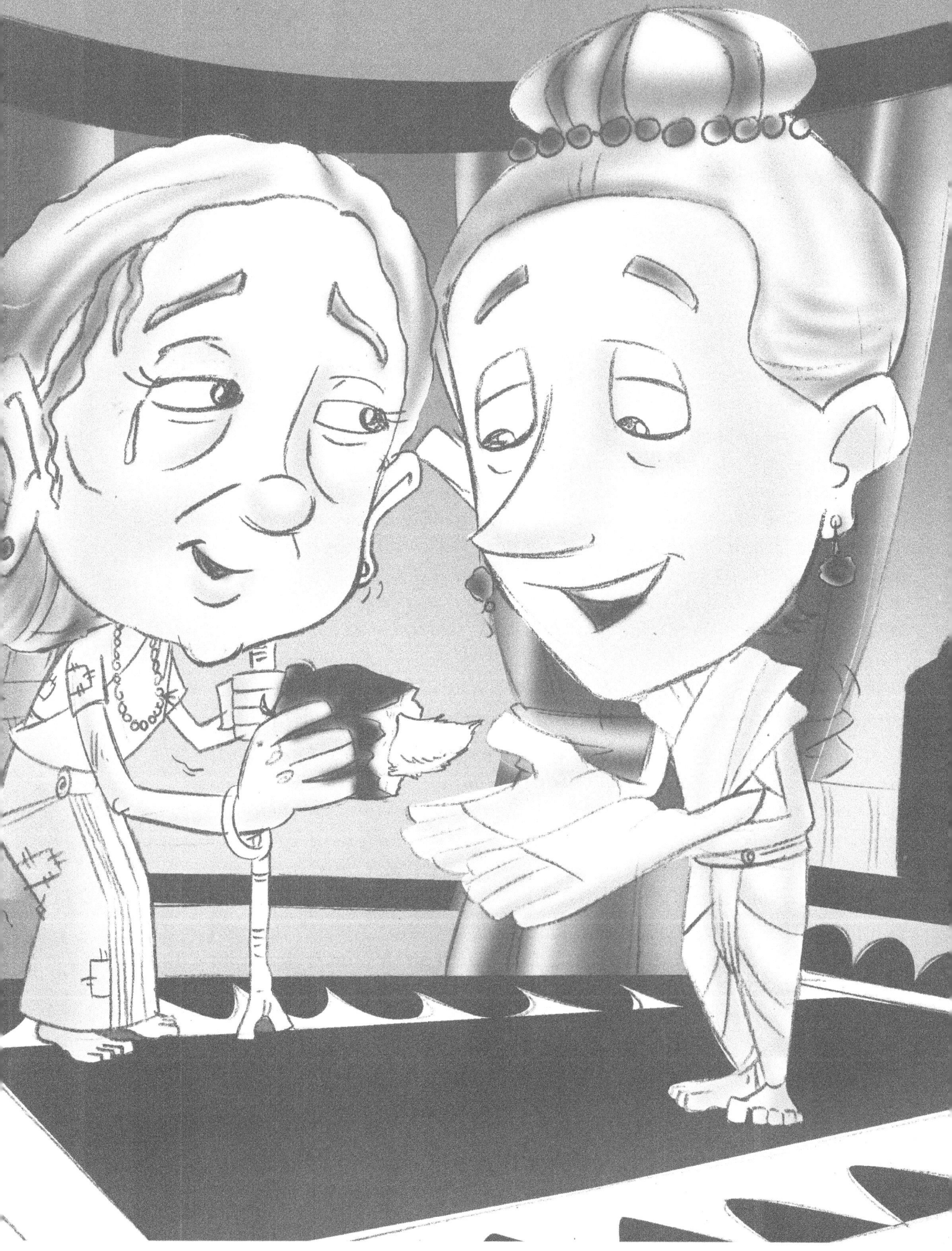

the biggest charity

After a long time Gautam Budha decided to proceed from the capital of Magadh. When citizens of Magadh got to know that Lord Buddha was leaving their city they went to meet him one final time with their offerings. And king Bimbisar also arrived there with his precious offerings. To accept all offerings Buddha was raising his right hand a little as a sign of acceptance. In the gathering of thousands of people an old woman also came to give her final tribute to Buddha. When she met Buddha she spoke, 'Oh Lord! I am very poor I have nothing to give you in offering. I have found a fallen mango from the tree and that is what I would like you to have.' She placed the half eaten mango in front of Buddha which she herself has tasted.

To see half eaten mango Buddha asked, 'Mother! Where is the remaining half?' she replied, "I was eating this mango then the news of your departure reached to me. I have nothing to give to you other than this half eaten mango so I decided to bring it to you.' Buddha came down from his seat and spread his both hands in order to accept the old woman's offering of half eaten mango.

King Bimbisar was astounded and asked Lord Buddha, 'Lord! You have accepted the most valuable gifts as part of your offerings with the gesture of one hand but to accept the old woman's half eaten mango you came down from your thrown. What is so peculiar about her mango?'

Buddha replied, 'whatever you all have offered me is only a small part of you people's income. You people bear a trace of pride in your hearts for doing charity. Whereas this old woman had nothing to give other than a half-eaten mango as part of the offering. She has with great devotion and un-selfish desire has given me whatever she had even then she has softness and love visible on her face.'

Moral

Any charity done with selflessness and love is the biggest act of any kind.

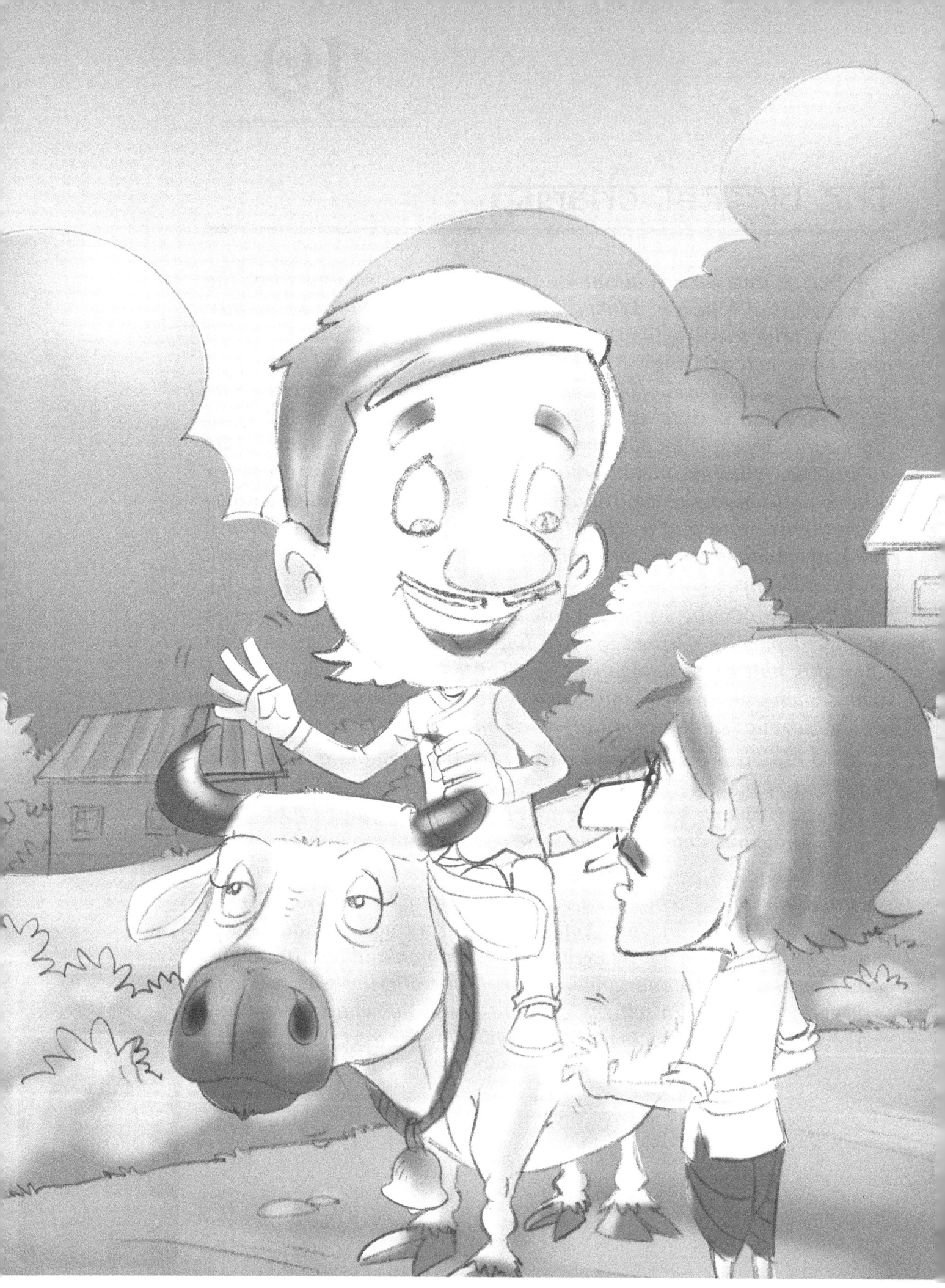

happiness

*O*ne day Mohan Lal was wearing a thick coat; he was tying a rope on his waste and was roaming from one point to the other sitting on his bull. Suddenly he started playing his flute. One pedestrian asked him, 'Brother! Why are you so happy? Did you get some treasure today?' Mohanlal said 'you can think like this. The real reason behind my happiness is not less than a real treasure.'

The pedestrian asked again. 'What the real reason? You could tell me as well.' Mohanlal said 'First reason is I am a human being and can enjoy several objects which are made for human usage only. Second is I am a male therefore I can appreciate God's best and most beautiful creation which is woman. The third reason is now that I have grown old and have conquered a lot of knowledge by living life till a ripe age and I have lived longer that those who lost their lives at an early age, now I have seen the whole world. And forth reason is I am ready to face the death because I have no fear or worry.' Then the pedestrian spoke 'you are right brother, a man who has found the right reason to spend his life fully does not need any other thing because such a person has nothing to worry not even death.'

The way Mohan Lal had lived his life was akin to his having wipe away every tear from the eyes of people he met for him death shall be no more, neither shall be suffer any morning, nor crying, nor pain anymore for all these things have passed away from his life.

Moral

To think & perceive life's happiness everyone has their own opinion. How happy or worried one is depends on their approach towards it.

STUDENT DEVELOPMENT/LEARNING

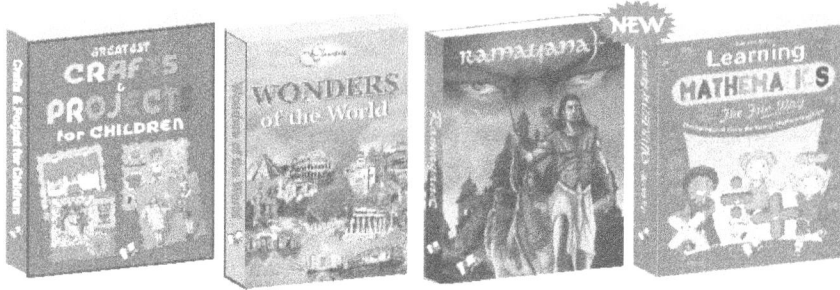

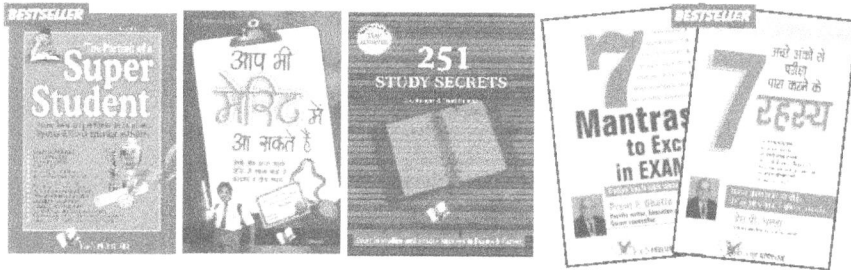

POPULAR SCIENCE

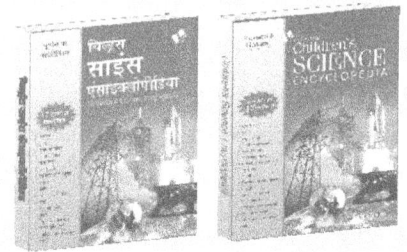

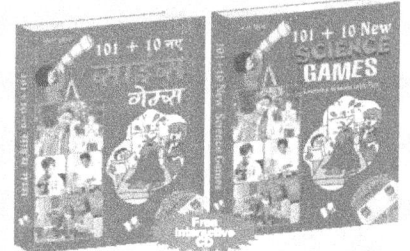

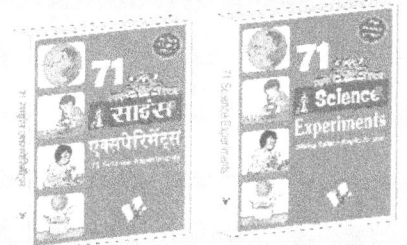

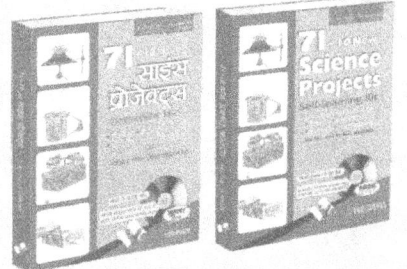

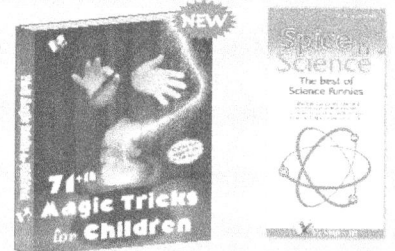

PUZZLES

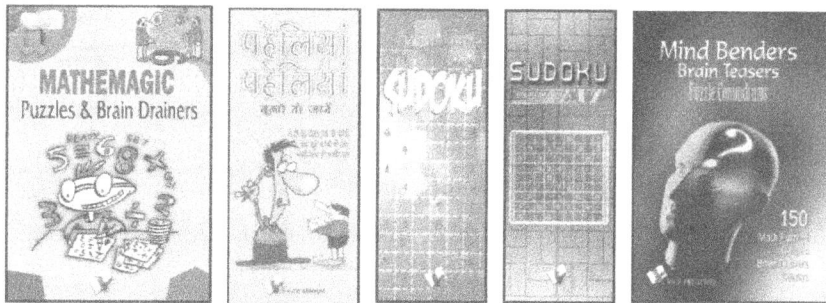

DRAWING BOOKS

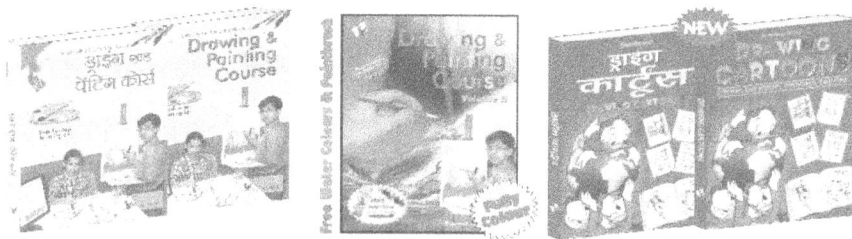

VALUE PACKS

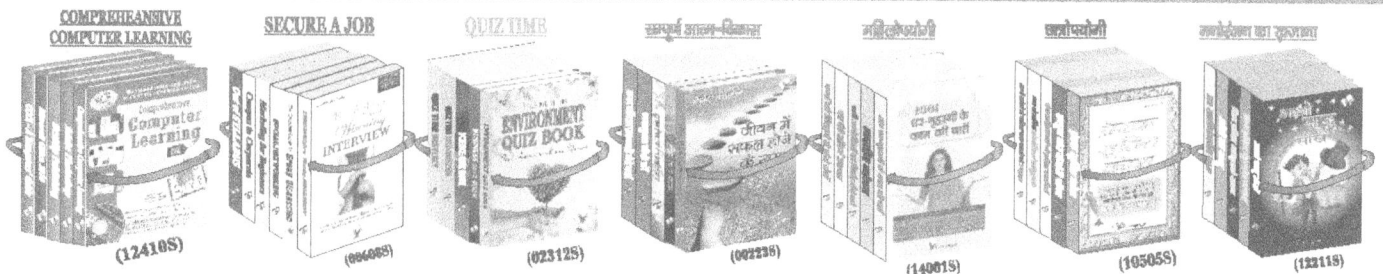

All books available at **www.vspublishers.com**

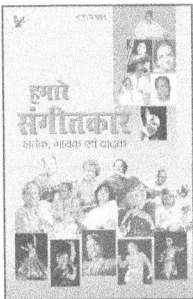

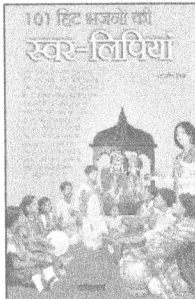

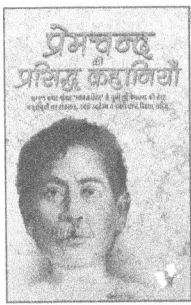

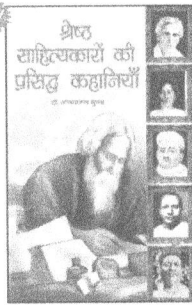

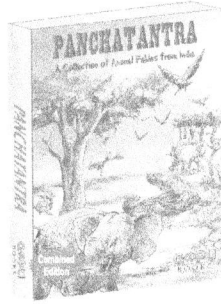

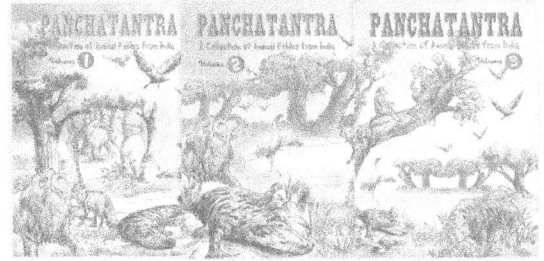

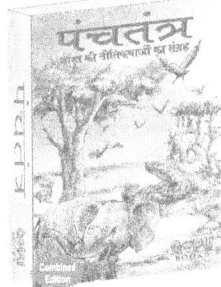

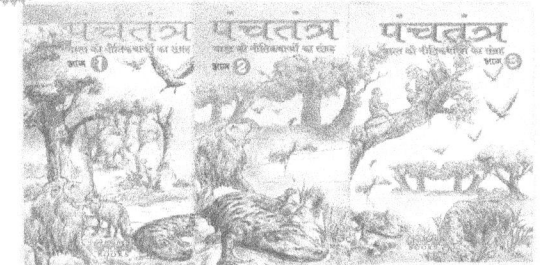

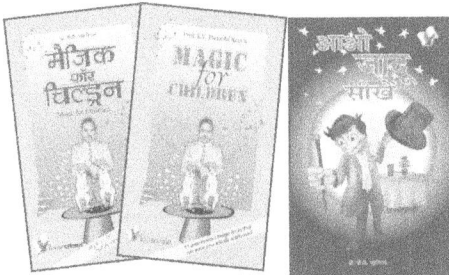

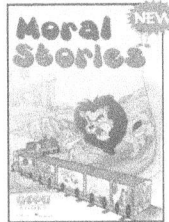

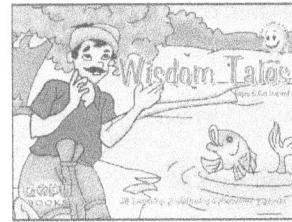

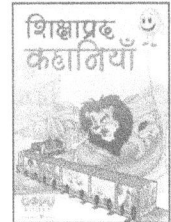

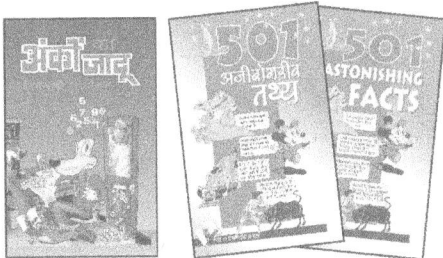

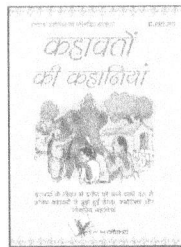

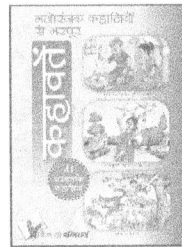

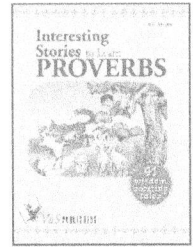

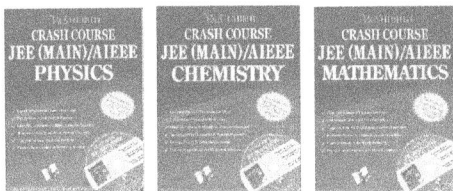

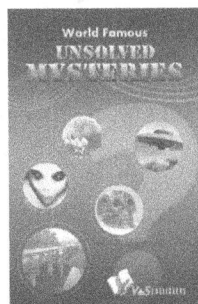

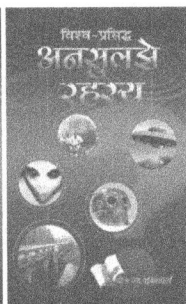

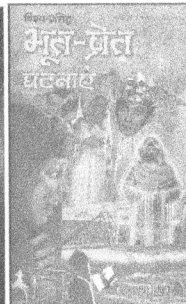

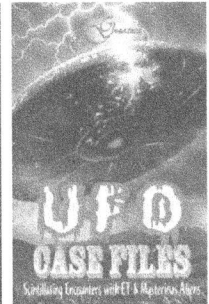

www.ingramcontent.com/pod-product-compliance
Lightning Source LLC
Chambersburg PA
CBHW080243270326
41926CB00020B/4357